The Dying Body as a Lived Experience

The anxiety over death persists in everyday life—though often denied or repressed—lingering as an unconscious worry or intuition that typically seems to compromise one's feelings of well-being and experience in a range of areas; coming out often as malaise, depression, and anger in much conduct. If one accepts the cliché that life is preparation for death, we must accept that the lived experience of the dying body is not highlighted merely in obvious cases of deterioration, such as in the aging or diseased body, but in everyday life as a normal phenomenon.

This book proposes that sensitivity to this dimension can empower us to develop creative relationships to the vulnerability of others and to ourselves as well. Part I lays the groundwork for a study of the ways the aura and fear of death recurs as a constant premonition in life and how people try to deal with this uneasiness. Part II then goes on to apply this focus to particular concerns and problems such as dementia, depression, aging, retirement, and a range of anxieties, frustrations, and aggressions.

The Dying Body as a Lived Experience will be of interest to a wide interdisciplinary audience in the health sciences, in the sociology of health and illness, philosophy, bioethics, and in the expanding field of medical humanities.

Alan Blum is Executive Director of the Culture of Cities Centre and Senior Professor of Sociology and Communication and Culture at York University, Canada. He is the author of *The Grey Zone of Health and Illness*, *Theorizing*, and the *Imaginative Structure of the City*, and co-author of *On the Beginning of Social Inquiry* and *Self-Reflection in the Arts and Sciences*.

Routledge Studies in the Sociology of Health and Illness

Available titles include:

Dimensions of Pain
Humanities and Social Science Perspectives
Edited by Lisa Folkmarson Käll

Aging Men, Masculinities and Modern Medicine
Edited by Antje Kampf, Barbara L. Marshall and Alan Petersen

Disclosure in Health and Illness
Mark Davis and Lenore Manderson

Caring and Well-being
A Lifeworld Approach
Kathleen Galvin and Les Todres

Systems Theory and the Sociology of Health and Illness
Observing Healthcare
Edited by Morten Knudsen and Werner Vogd

Complaints, Controversies and Grievances in Medicine
Edited by Jonathan Reinarz and Rebecca Wynter

The Public Shaping of Medical Research
Patient Associations, Health Movements and Biomedicine
Edited by Peter Wehling and Willy Viehöver

Giving Blood
The Institutional Making of Altruism
Edited by Johanne Charbonneau and André Smith

Health, Food and Social Inequality
Critical Perspectives on the Supply and Marketing of Food
Carolyn Mahoney

Forthcoming titles:

Vaginal Examination in Labour
Challenging contemporary practice
Mary Stewart

Transnationalising Reproduction
Third Party Conception in a Globalised World
Edited by Roisin Ryan Flood and Jenny Gunnarsson Payne

The Social Determinants of Male Health
John MacDonald

Fathering Children with Autism

Needs, Practices and Service Use
Carol Potter

Socio-economics of Personalized Medicine in Asia
Shirley Hsiao-Li Sun

Financing Healthcare in China
Towards universal health insurance
Sabrina Ching Yuen Luk

The Dying Body as a Lived Experience

Alan Blum

Routledge
Taylor & Francis Group
LONDON AND NEW YORK

First published 2017 by Routledge

2 Park Square, Milton Park, Abingdon, Oxfordshire OX14 4RN
52 Vanderbilt Avenue, New York, NY 10017

Routledge is an imprint of the Taylor & Francis Group, an informa business

First issued in paperback 2019

British Library Cataloguing-in-Publication Data
A catalogue record for this book is available from the British Library

Library of Congress Cataloging in Publication Data
Names: Blum, Alan, 1935- , author.
Title: The dying body as lived experience / Alan Blum.
Other titles: Routledge studies in the sociology of health and illness.
Description: Abingdon, Oxon ; New York, NY : Routledge, 2017. |
Series: Routledge studies in the sociology of health and illness | Includes bibliographical references and index.
Identifiers: LCCN 2016013501| ISBN 9781138655157 (hardback) | ISBN 9781315622712 (ebook)
Subjects: | MESH: Attitude to Death | Anxiety | Dementia | Philosophy
Classification: LCC BF789.D4 | NLM BF 789.D4 | DDC 155.9/37--dc23
LC record available at http://lccn.loc.gov/2016013501

ISBN: 978-1-138-65515-7 (hbk)
ISBN: 978-0-367-22404-2 (pbk)

Typeset in Times New Roman
by Saxon Graphics Ltd, Derby

The author and publisher are pleased to acknowledge the support of the Faculty of Liberal Arts & Professional Studies, York University, Toronto, Canada

Contents

Acknowledgments

As an author of a book on death and dying during these years, no matter how hard I try to be sentient, scintillating and sexy, I know that I cannot have been a comforting presence for family, friends, and intimates during this period of writing. I first will try to repair such a baleful influence by affirming the steadfast support of my creative and accomplished wife Elke Grenzer whose good sense and flexibility in the face of a turbulent presence such as mine graced these years by constantly inspiring me to interrupt my obsession and to reflect upon living rather than dying by reminding me forcefully and eloquently how I might fail at one while succeeding at the other. Elke doesn't know it and might not believe it, but she has truly been my muse. Despite the possible reservations they might have towards my paternal finesse, I reiterate that my three engaging daughters Paula, Beth and Hannah showed me in their different ways how living in the present must comprehend and try to sustain the dreams and vitality that they have shown me and in these ways allowed me to enjoy them and what they promise to do with their lives. I found their relations to creativity enabling in different ways. I have not always been artful in expressing my feelings towards them and like Lear only want them to acknowledge that their dad mattered (LOL!!!). I treasure the humour and ingenuity of Beth's talented husband Jean-Christophe Cloutier whose relationship to me has always been generous, enjoyable and thought-provoking.

Good friends come to mind such as the Bonners, both Margaret and Kieran, who have engaged and nurtured me over the years with sympathy and intellectual vitality, and even more, with a sustained jouissance that enabled us often to laugh and play together as creative and not moribund souls. The reliability of Stanley Raffel and his capacity to mix and match syllogism and metaphor in his work has been important for me over the years in many ways. I have always learned from my encounters and friendship with Paddy Colfer, and from workshops of the Culture of Cities Centre and its many valuable practitioners who are too numerous to mention as the cliché goes but must include the ever provocative Steve Bailey, Saeed Hydaralli's constant efforts to put his thought to test, and such recent and friendly students such as Celia Huang and Benjamin Waterman. The reawakening of relationships with David Lynes and dear, dedicated Andreani Papadopolou, especially in workshops in Greece, always energized me by pointing to the relevance of nurturing experiences of the past and expectations for the future not only as indications of loyalty but as essential to the continuity of the quality of work and the dream of community. In recent years It has been my good fortune to attract the talented and most intelligent Han Zhang as a graduate student whose dissertation research encouraged me to try to digest the influences of China in my own work and to work with her to sort out the complex problem of the aged under contemporary conditions.

Tangible influences include of course agencies such as the Social Sciences and Humanities Research Council of Canada that has funded many of the projects in which I was involved, the Canadian Institutes of Health Research whose funding enabled me to begin research on health and dementia, and intermittently the University of Waterloo. My home base York University has offered me support in different ways and most recently in permitting me the services of the excellent graduate student Leigh Denholm who has helped so much in preparing this manuscript. I thank Penni Stewart and Phil Walsh who have helped me of late negotiate the bureaucratic terrain of this university.

In very recent years three special collaborations come to mind: Bruce Janz of the University of Central Florida has encouraged my work from his perspective as a philosopher with acumen and sympathy; I have collaborated in recent work with Stuart Murray of Carleton University who has influenced me to treat his good nature and critical sensibilities as the model for an innovative impulse in the present climate; finally, the generosity and intellectual breadth of Barry Sandywell starting from the old days in London England, reflected in his responsiveness to my work and to me as a person as well, has so revived me in recent years that I readily accepted his suggestion for the title of this book.

The danger of acknowledgments is that they can become like interminable academy award speeches but a book on death and dying has to risk being somewhat obsessive about memory and influences although this could read like a prospective obituary. So an acknowledgment such as this must tread the thin line drawn by this impasse without either melting or continuing indefinitely. The problem of being eloquent and not shameless in writing about oneself seems to be a challenge for stand-up comedy.

Prologue
The Dying Body as a Lived Experience

In Sophocles' play, *Oedipus at Colonus*, the chorus says that not to be born may be the greatest boon of all, raising the eternal question of the meaning of such an enigmatic declaration. If we check online reactions to this statement we see that it tends to be treated as an empirical proposition that is argued about with vehemence as true or false whereas I take Sophocles to use it as the sign of an impasse, an opening that we need to take up as an invitation to inquire into a question that we might never settle conclusively but still need to engage. Certainly life as a living experience requires knowledge and the oriented sentience and reflection we identify with knowing as necessary but knowledge brings with it in the words of Benardete's restatement of the chorus "murder, civil fractions, strife, battles, and jealous resentment" (Benardete 2000, 114). That knowledge brings both good and evil, the Grey Zone, means that not to be born, though unimaginable, must be without knowledge, raising the question of whether life is worth the price. This book opens up a path into this question and the impossibility of an answer as itself the sign of the most fundamental impasse. Implicitly this book raises the question of whether asking about what cannot be answered is worth the price, is worth writing about or whether it is better not to write this book than to write it at all, here echoing a reviewer's words about the novelist John Barth and some others if "after so many books about death, there is a story beyond biological decline that will sustain … (the) … imagination" (Burn 2008, 20).

This book addresses ways in which the aura of death haunts everyday life as a tacit, unsettling but forceful awareness of mortality, a reminder of limits much like the "foreign intruder" Laplanche used to identify the unconscious and its "message" (1976). I focus on the effects of the premonition of mortality on lived experience as an implicit source of anxiety, neither simply bodily nor cognitive, but affective at its core and linked to a sense of the fundamental ambiguity of human existence in time and the persistent lure of melancholy evoked by an apprehension of the abandonment of meaning.

My title appropriates the notion of the "lived experience" from phenomenology that is typically used to make reference to the experience of a living being and implies that such an experience has to be oriented to in ways that include death as part of life. This not only accepts the cliché that life is preparation for death, that we live in a way that inevitably must move toward such an end, but also that this experience is not highlighted merely in obvious cases of deterioration, such as in the aging or diseased body that might still live in a resigned way, but in everyday life as a normal phenomenon.

Although anxiety around the premonition of death has haunted philosophy and art over time both in the west and Asia, the book seeks to engage as its primary question the problem of the ways in which the experience of modernity has been represented as influencing this anxiety over death. Such influences appear in a canon after Plato in works of those such as Hegel, Benjamin, Heidegger, Lacan, and many others who engage death in various ways. Consequently, the problem of suffering embodiment is a central focus as described and exemplified in a canon. Yet, in addition to this canon, the phenomenon of collective death is a significant dimension and horizon of the modern era, as discussed for example in Edith Wyschogrod's book, *Spirit in Ashes: Hegel, Heidegger, and Man-Made Mass Death*, which explores the form of life of what she calls the "death-event" and "death-world" of mass, industrial-technical extermination, and its shaping power over our conceptions of living, self, temporality, and language (1985). Finally, the technological advances of mass media that have resulted in the worldwide dissemination of information and representations of death in many shapes besides broadcasting the news seems to produce a unique exposure to the fact of death and to its normalization and particular character in different guises in the fine arts and specifically in the novel.

Thus, a discourse on suffering as expressed in a collective speech that I typify after Durkheim as a Writing Machine must be both a topic and resource of and for this work. The Writing Machine includes besides the canon, literature on atrocities and catastrophes such as the Holocaust and extremist purges, survivor testimony, collective trauma, the escalation of the "death event" in the Cold War, and the spectre of the ultimate threat of total death/nuclear war/etc. Yet the writing of society in the shape of its news, reports, obituaries, and tolls, monuments, and archives of the dead, must also include the representations of fiction and literature that seek always to wrestle from finite characterizations, reports, and descriptions, some sense of the infinite and particular experience of suffering embodiment and its ambiguity. Accordingly, I seek to explicate ways in which this voice of otherness is articulated in popular culture, film, literature, social theory, and philosophy through its materialization in ethical collisions that make reference to such thematic issues.

In my project, the foreign intruder is the resonance of death itself as it is reflected in various illustrations both mundane and dramatic. For example, besides coming to view in debates over issues such as organ donation, the death penalty, informed consent, care giving in dementia, and the attribution of responsibility for crimes and atrocities that recur in typical representations of both survivors and perpetrators, the foreign intruder is implicit in many guises such as "normal" loneliness, demoralization, desperation, settings of rehabilitation, and propensities for acting-out on many occasions. My book intends to penetrate and lay out such mundane (dis)guises of anxiety over mortality in a number of different cases including both these "normal" situations, and the issues and debates just mentioned here, and additionally on occasion in films depicting characters "falling apart," and in works of selected novelists such as Anita Brookner, Thomas Bernhard, Hans Keilson, James Salter, Miriam Toews, Virginia Woolf, and others who portray a subject fascinated by the refrain of *Memento Mori* in various circumstances and motivated by the spell it seems to cast (see particularly the various studies of Suzanne England and especially 2015).

References

Benardete, Seth. 2000. "On Greek Tragedy." In *The Argument of the Action: Essays on Greek Poetry and Philosophy*, 99–145. Chicago: University of Chicago Press.

Burn, Stephen. 2008. "'Much adieu': Review of J. Barth, The Development." Pg. 20 in *Times Literary Supplement*, October 17 2008.

England, Suzanne. 2015. "Moral Complexities in Old Age in Muriel Spark's *Momento Mori,*" *Journal of Aging Studies* 33: 76–85.

Laplanche, Jean. (1970) 1976. *Life and Death in Psychoanalysis*. Translated by Jeffrey Mehlman. Baltimore: Johns Hopkins University Press.

Wyschogrod, Edith. 1985. *Spirit in Ashes: Hegel, Heidegger, and Man-Made Mass Death*. New Haven: Yale University Press.

Introduction

Living Life and Forgetting Death

Émile Durkheim suggests that the very fact that most people live seems as if a choice to live, not particularly reflective and oriented but somewhat as an automated occurrence similar to what Lacan has described as drive. From this angle, the desire to live reveals desire as a kind of forceful insistence, almost corporeal, that compels us to continue at life despite particular inclinations. That life seems not a choice (except when it is noticed as oriented, as in exceptional circumstances, acts of violence, or suicide) shows its similarity to many habits or routines that Simmel identifies as unexceptional until infractions occur (e.g. mistakes, or infelicities in logic, or in customs such as greetings that are noticed when they are absent but otherwise disregarded). This is to say that the desire to continue at life is not noticed unless it is made a spectacle through infraction or exceptional circumstances. Simmel's conception of our conduct here makes reference to such an example not as rule following but as akin to automation as when he says that in such cases we do not "observe" the rule or treat a norm as an observance but carry it through unmindful of its constraint until an infraction or slippage occurs that makes it noticeable. Thus Simmel formulates such conduct as exemplary of what has been called adherence to the "seen-but-unnoticed" background expectancies that are accepted in ways that suspend concern for their conventionality by holding in abeyance such a regard as "uninteresting." Concerning such an oriented unmindfulness, I have suggested (for example in Blum 2011, 2014: 38) that continuing at life would be like this in contrast to Durkheim's comment on the continuation as a choice. At the end of *The Division of Labor* he remarks on how the fact that most people live displays a preference for life as if the choice, if it is a choice, is similar to an election result saying:

> The only experimental fact proving that life is generally good is that the great mass of men prefer it to death.
>
> (Durkheim [1893] 1933: 245)

So there are two suggestions here: the fact that we continue at life as an unreflected given, automated and habitual, or in Durkheim's sense, as indicative of a choice or commitment, in some way, to live.

Durkheim says:

> To be so, in the average life, happiness must prevail over unhappiness. If the relations were reversed, neither the attachment of men to life, nor its continuance jostled by the facts at each moment could be understood. Pessimists … explain the persistence of this phenomenon by the illusions of hope. According to them, if … we hold onto life, it is because we are wrongly hoping that the future will make up for the past. But … hope … does not explain itself. It has not miraculously descended from heaven into our hearts, but it has had to be formed, as all sentiments, within the action of the facts. If … men have learned to hope … they have acquired the habit of turning their eyes toward the future, and of awaiting compensations for their present sufferings.
>
> ([1893] 1933, 245)

The implication of Durkheim's recognition for a conception of life is that it is not chosen but still must reflect a need and desire that discloses life and all of its mundane things as casting a lure upon us as the spell of our automation. Here, the spell is identified as materializing in perseverance, habituation, and routines that seem to the spellbound subject as if chosen, but can only be a result of sources that remain inexplicable. In this view Christianity might affirm that the mystery of creation manifests itself in the inscrutable causal enigma of any innocuous action. The subject seems in this view as an automaton, living out routines as if under the spell of sociality in the shape of codes and a normative order. The automated tone of the human condition, its repetitive and compulsory commitment to doing as it does and must do, seems not only to account for life itself but for many of the devices and technologies that we develop for living as in our customs, language, and formulae, and even the interpretive constructions and models we use to represent "reality" as in the invention of codes and clichés that we honor.

René Girard (1977) affirms that the myth of spontaneous desire masks the mimetic relationship we accept as our basic inheritance regardless of how fiercely we champion our voluntarism. The automated character of human existence, this relentlessness of drive, gives Mario Perniola cause to speak of addiction as the exemplary model of desire today (2004). What this suggests is that the driven human subject seems to exemplify the commitment to life as addictive, making relations to life conceivable as postures (or strategies) for handling addiction. From this view, life is problem-solving in the way that an addiction seems to illustrate and in part we handle the "problem" of living by developing performance-enhancing drugs. So Durkheim and Simmel can be seen to converge in their conception of the continuance at life as automated conduct that is not reflective of choice or preference in the conventional sense but of the lure of automation itself as if an appeal that is in some way gripping. That life casts such a spell tells us something about the seen-but-unnoticed character of our "background" in between constraint and freedom as a zone of ambiguity that mixes compulsion and attraction, always suggesting that we seem connected to ourselves as both autonomous and self-affective intimate beings and as things subject to the force of automation.

Weber's Wrinkle: Abandonment—Anger, Betrayal, Acting-Out

Part of the lure of automation as the fascination with our own mechanistic potential was supported by the belief that we could keep running because of the source of creation, inexplicable and trustworthy. In his *Protestant Ethic*, Weber claimed that ascetic Protestantism introduced the "withdrawal of the security and certainty of salvation," creating an analogue to Lacan's declaration that Other does not answer, as a problem-solving situation that asks how "in a world of irrevocable indeterminacy … does one establish his own indubitable value" (Blum 2003, 212)? If the solution that I called bourgeoisie there was simply to treat oneself as chosen and as bearer of self-worth by virtue of that, it not only fits Simmel's formula for seeing the typical uninteresting reflexive character of life itself for the mass, but captures Gadamer's notion of the primordial repression bequeathed by Prometheus to humans, the capacity to forget death.

Now though, Freud and Bataille become interesting interruptions in this discourse and provocative interlocutors. Just as Freud's conception of mourning and melancholia identifies the sadness and anger that must invariably result from such abandonment, Bataille formulates such a response as a reaction to betrayal as if life had affirmed its priority and eternality all along as a deceit that is at some point uncovered and recognized as the lie that it was and is. The problem then becomes one of having to deal with the anger and sadness that ensues from the abandonment of meaning and the inevitable melancholic sense of helplessness and hopelessness. Girard has described this as a sacrificial crisis that can only motivate us to direct our anger for the betrayal to the source imagined as responsible, the source typically viewed as the agent seeming responsible for the withdrawal of the assurance of salvation. As a problem-solving situation, then, we recognize the need for a target or for objects on which we can displace our frustration.

> Having said that there is one thing that man hasn't managed to come to terms with and that is death, the Chorus says that he has come up with an absolutely marvelous gimmick, namely translated literally, "an escape into impossible sicknesses."… He hasn't managed to come to terms with death but he invents marvelous gimmicks in the form of sicknesses he himself fabricates. There is something extraordinary about finding that notion expressed in 441 B.C. as one of mankind's essential dimensions. It wouldn't make any sense to translate that as "an escape from sicknesses." … That's quite a gimmick he has invented; make of it what you will.
>
> (Lacan [1959–1960] 1992, 275–276)

What we can make of this is that the sicknesses humans invent or fabricate are the many modes of adjustments or postures developed in response to the enigma of mortality. This is because the desire to overstep boundaries and towards excess endemic to our self-transcendence produces a great range of replies besides art and eros and theorizing, but repression, perversion, psychosis, including the myriad affects such as the longing and resignation noted by Simmel. Care then is in part "produced" by the sicknesses fabricated by humans in trying to solve the impossible problem of mortality and in this way makes everyone a potential recipient of care and everyone, at their best, a potential caregiver.

In this sense both depression and anger would be examples of such "gimmicks" insofar as they are socially constructed paths of escape or "adjustments" to the experience of mortality as a burden. For example, in Annie Baker's play, *The Flick*, a character identifies his depression as an intended solution to his perpetual experience of disappointment in life, revealing such a sickness as a gimmick in Lacan's sense not as a sign of duplicity but as if a solution to a problem that any symptom can be seen to exhibit (Baker, 2014).

As I write this, a celebrity entertainer in the US, a popular comedian named Robin Williams, has committed suicide and the immediate responses to this act in mass media bear scrutiny in relation to my topic (see Hawksworth 2014; Lenti 2014; *The Huffington Post Canada* 2014). The reactions to Williams' death, at many levels, reveal an interpretive relationship to death in the collective as part of its ways and means of conceiving of dying and the kinds of issues its consideration raises for the question of life. At the extremes, suicide seems to respondents to disclose weakness or strength of will, a cowardly decision or, in contrast, a heroic plunge into darkness. Two points seem constant in this interpretive structure: first, that suicide is and was a "decision," and second that such a decision, whatever its "cause," symptomatizes depression and certainly something called "mental illness." Thus, the respondents who argue that suicide shows an "awful weakness" are counteracted by those who contend that it "takes an incredible amount of strength" (a rare point of view) or, typically, that it results from a "disease" or feeling of desperation. The mass of respondents cannot understand suicide as an encounter with the meaning of life in relation to mortality and tend to view it as weakness, craziness, and—at worst—selfishness in "giving up on life." Whereas the more sophisticated responses tend to medicalize suicide by seeing it as depression and mental illness, at the other extreme, it is regarded as an inability to suffer the reduced lifestyle that "drinks lemonade rather than champagne." All do seem to recognize that suicide as a decision against life reveals a loss of pleasure and a pronounced inability to administer the jouissance demanded of living with the "real" demands of life. Whether the subject is seen as weak, selfish, or a victim of deranged pathos, the enigmatic sources of the action cause many to be reflective about the meaning of life, suggesting that it requires endurance, patience, and self-control because "many people out there" are believed to suffer mental illness and depression as part of their inability to measure up to these demands. With the exception of those most primitive responses that search for concrete causes in financial trouble or particular types of external critical moments, the more enlightened identify mental illness as a mysterious force, most likely of corporeal nature, that insists itself upon the weak and unfortunate souls who always remain in some way vulnerable to life's stresses and strains.

In this work, I include such responses as part of the writing of society, or what I call its Writing Machine, as a way of tracking the collective relationship to the life of dying and conceptions of mortality. This pursuit invites me to attempt to penetrate this collection of opinions and beliefs as if it is a surface of many indications concerning life, its limits and ambiguity, and to consider how we might imagine stronger relations to living than riding a roller coaster of fluctuations in frustrations, as if we inhabit the seat of a passenger either too weak or insufficiently strong to endure the ride. This allows me to consider suicide too, as one particular way of engaging this, neither as weak nor strong, but as a relationship to problem-solving in a situation where the problem is the irresolution with which we are constantly confronted. Thus, instead of relying on labels such as depression or mental illness, or easy appeals to corporeal disintegration, I will consider desperation as what Durkheim calls a normal social fact and an opportunity for theorizing, research, and hopefully, healing. In this work, I begin to theorize death as an elementary social phenomenon that dramatizes the question of meaning, and its aesthetic and ethical registers, that is persistently blocked, repressed, or fetishized in the normal run of affairs. I proceed by developing a relation between death and what I call the Grey Zone or fundamental ambiguity of language and action.

Now we can make clear the status of Durkheim's proposition and the hypothetical dialogue I see it as sustaining with Simmel, for what is raised is the question: what does it mean to live? Both Durkheim and Simmel remove life from its position as a site of innate value, seeing it in its way as beyond good and evil and so as a condition that can or cannot be invested with value. That life reveals no choice but simply a kind of thrownness in the idiom of Heidegger, causes us to consider the everlasting refrain, is it a gift given or a punishment that is dispensed, and so, what must we make of it? This question places death as a paradigm of the human condition not because of its hermeneutic mysteries but because it represents the *sine qua non* of a condition, an inheritance, that invites us to act, to make something out of a mute signifier by giving it meaning and so, by showing the acceptance this requires. Death as the paradigm of the condition (applicable in its way as a model for any condition such as gender, age, race, or class), discloses the condition first as beyond good or evil, and most important, as the indifferent circumstance that frames all action by compelling us to make such an inheritance choice-worthy.

According to Blond, this is the problem Rosenzweig formulated: "The task of human beings is to persevere and find endurance in a world always already perishing." (Blond 2010, 53) Accordingly, what Rosenzweig spoke of as the need of love to conquer death, a need intuited through what he called revelation, can be understood as a need to accept and be committed to the present, to reject the linear or timeless time as he called it. To make life choice-worthy presupposes reflecting on how we might contribute to life by rethinking in this way, the question of what value life can be said to have and to what life does contribute. This reflection assumes that we can imagine the absence or otherness of life, the limit upon it that leads us to explore Plato's query on how something is unlike what is other to it and in this case, how life is unlike what is other to it. This invites us to imagine the otherness that is unlike life by engaging the abyss of Non-Being that we can only fantasize. This is how we can say that a hallucination or delusion must underlie all meaning.

References

Baker, Annie. 2014. *The Flick.* New York: Theatre Communication Group.

Bataille, Georges. (1973) 1989. *Theory of Religion.* Translated by Robert Hurley. New York: Zone Books.

Blond, Louis P. 2010. "Franz Rosenzweig: Homelessness in Time." *New German Critique* 111: 27–58.

Blum, Alan. 2003. *The Imaginative Structure of the City.* Montreal: McGill-Queen's University Press.

——. 2011. "Life, Death, and the In-Between: The Duck-Rabbit/The Face of the Clown." In Tristanne Connolly (ed.), *Spectacular Death: Interdisciplinary Perspectives on Morality and (Un)representability.* Bristol: Intellect, pp. 21–42.

——. 2014. "Durkheim's Ruse: The Concept as a Seduction." *Canadian Journal of Sociology* 39(4): 38.

De Coulanges, Fustel. (1864) 1955. *The Ancient City.* New York: Doubleday Anchor

Durkheim, Émile. (1893) 1933. *The Division of Labor in Society.* Translated by George Simpson. New York: The Free Press.

Gadamer, Hans-Georg. (1993) 1996. *The Enigma of Health: The Art of Healing in a Scientific Age.* Translated by John Gaiger and Nicholas Walker. Stanford: Stanford University Press.

Girard, René. (1972) 1977. *Violence and the Sacred.* Translated by Patrick Gregory. Baltimore: Johns Hopkins University Press.

Hawksworth, Elizabeth. 2014. "Don't Call Robin Williams' Death a Waste." *The Huffington Post Canada*, August 12. Available at: www.huffingtonpost.ca/elizabeth-hawksworth/robin-williams-suicide_b_5670205.html. Last accessed September 27, 2014.

The Huffington Post Canada. 2014. "Toronto Star Slammed for 'Insensitive' Robin Williams Tweet." *The Huffington Post Canada*, August 12. Available at: www.huffingtonpost.ca/2014/08/12/robin-williams-toronto-star-tweet_n_5672521.html. Last accessed September 27, 2014.

Lacan, Jacques. (1959–1960) 1992. *The Seminar of Jacques Lacan, Book VII: The Ethics of Psychoanalysis 1959–1960.* Edited by Jacques-Alain Miller. Translated by Dennis Porter. New York: Norton.

Lenti, Erica. 2014. "Williams' Death Makes Me Think of Myself Back on the Edge of that Subway Platform." *The Huffington Post Canada*, August 12. Available at: www.huffingtonpost.ca/erica-lenti/robin-williams-suicide_b_5672255.html. Last accessed September 27, 2014.

Perniola, Mario. (2000) 2004. *The Sex Appeal of the Inorganic: Philosophies of Desire in the Modern World.* Translated by Massimo Verdicchio. New York and London: Continuum.

Weber, Max. (1905) 1930. *The Protestant Ethic and the Spirit of Capitalism.* Translated by Talcott Parsons. London: George Allen & Unwin.

Part I

Death, Mystery, Life

> Death was the first mystery, and it placed man on the track of other mysteries. It raised his thoughts from the visible to the invisible, from the transitory to the eternal, from the human to the divine.
>
> (de Coulanges [1864] 1955, 25)

In his primordial rhapsody to death, Fustel de Coulanges considers it the event that stimulates humans to engage the perplexity of existence, and so, as an incentive to thought that needs to reflect upon its conditions and limits. We might treat this as an ontological view that glosses the anxiety and paralysis of thought-thinking itself that it covers over, leading us to appreciate a more dialectical engagement with death, with the tension between its pleasure in promising to relieve us of worldly turmoil, and its pain in forcing us to inhabit a zone of ambiguity and trepidation, as a mix that seems to originate not in intellect, choice, or will but as a kind of force that grips us all as if a spell cast upon us that seems universal (happening to everyone), particular (happening to oneself in a way that is unshareable), and without rhyme or reason that could give satisfaction.

Gadamer among others ([1993] 1996, 156) tells us that the gift of Prometheus to humankind for which Zeus punished him was not fire, as typically thought, but the capacity to forget death. This gift was developed by Aeschylus' reading of the myth.

> The myth relates how Prometheus stole fire from heaven and taught mankind to work with it. But Aeschylus presents the story in a way which makes the theft of fire almost incidental. Prometheus glories in having performed the greatest possible service to man—who had been left so poor and defenseless by Zeus—by depriving him of the knowledge of his own death.

Amnesia is a peculiar gift, and it confirms Lucretius, who would smile wisely and say "of course!" The truth is sacrificed and humans need to live with false beliefs in order to survive. The truth would kill them, annihilate their spirit. As Deleuze says, nihilism is the loss of a belief in life, and so, the primordial repression of death is the human way of silencing the voice of nihilism.

Bataille ([1973] 1989, 51), quite a different character than Gadamer, agrees in his idiomatic way.

> The anxiousness to remain personally alive that establishes the person's individuality is linked to the integration of existence into the world of things … work and the fear of dying are interdependent … man is an individual to the extent that his apprehension ties him to the results of labor.

If death is forgotten as if a truth to be discarded, this gesture of forgetting can take many shapes, for example, discussed by Freud and Lacan as the repression that Gadamer mentions, or as disavowal that simply rejects the truth, or finally as foreclosure that ceases to speak about it as if its truth, conceded in a sense, is unspeakable. Bataille intimates that the first shape of repression lies in work, productivity, and what we might call the preoccupation of humans with worldly pursuits and things. This shape of forgetting death we can call *bourgeoisie*. That our being occupied by things means in its way that the disturbing character of death is displaced and channeled into some notion of our productivity that is designed to affirm our extension in some way, that our end is only apparent because we will continue to live in our labor and its effects. It has been noted that children are treated in such ways to affirm the fertility of unending heterosexuality.

Bataille identifies such a repression as a betrayal of sorts made transparent when we are cut off from our preoccupations. For example, leisure, retirement, free time or time freed from preoccupation, all can bring us face-to-face with the point of life. Or being without family or relationship (to paraphrase a character in the movie *Grand Hotel*, "a man without a woman is a dead man," we can translate in a less sexist way "a person without another is a dead duck!") bringing together under the cloak of idleness the retired, single, unemployed, and even the flâneur, as icons of isolation detached from preoccupation, or condemned to being preoccupied with self alone. Thus, if work is one way of repressing death, we see that death always returns to haunt the working life in the shape of free time, but more directly in the collective fascination with the thing itself, its superfluity and lack of intimacy. This is how the repression that is bourgeoisie is always exercised by the aura of the alienation it senses as a riveting focus of attention in the superfluity of things (accounting for Plato's jab at the lovers of beautiful things who have given up loving beauty because it is a humanist illusion like any value). This sets up Bataille's notion that the immersion in things fears an encounter with intimacy (with the beauty of the thing).

1 Desperation as a Grey Zone

Introduction

The Grey Zone makes reference to the intellectual anxiety and hyperstimulation released by the typical and persistent aura of ambiguity that seems to inhabit our words and deeds as an unsettling constraint upon black-and-white judgment and action in any specific situation. As a figure of speech and not a specific area or region, the Grey Zone assumes many and diverse shapes as a trope that depicts a quality intrinsic rather than external to language, appearing in various guises from at least Asian antiquity and the parables and wisdom of the sages to current arts and sciences. The Grey Zone is then an interpretive landscape.

In images of "higher powers" in relation to mundanity, of Sun, River and such signs, in representations of Being and Nothing, finitude and infinity, faith and reason, in Kant's in-itself and Hegel's absolute, all the way through sense and reference, identity and predication, the unconscious, Empson's seven types of ambiguity and beyond, the Grey Zone in its various ways simply reiterates the truth of mediation and the fate of linguistic intermediacy, but is more too, for it testifies implicitly to the effects of such a fate upon the human actor, as one who must suffer such a condition, must orient to it in its convoluted and reduced shapes, and live under its auspices. This makes the Grey Zone something other than a metaphor for the polysemic aspects of language, as semiotics might have it, but akin to the Real as the fundamental ambiguity that we must suffer and negotiate in any circumstance, revealing that we are persistently subject to a remainder, to remains that are everlasting opportunities for other beginnings.

The Grey Zone is then a relationship or, in the idiom of sociology, a course of action. Philosophers I respect would refer to it as a concrete universal, meaning that any concept such as this has to materialize in action that is concrete and actual. In this way the abstraction of linguistic indeterminacy is necessarily translated and actualized in vital solutions and trajectories of problem-solving. Yet, as a relationship the Grey Zone most immediately comes to view in ordinary language as the space of ambiguity between one and another in interaction as the "noise" that complicates any model of a simple exchange (Serres [1991] 1997), say, as conceded in mistakes, infelicities, misrecognition, distortion and the like, this usage of noise itself tends to externalize "breakdown" as if it is simply a result of extraneous variables whereas the source of ambiguity much more deeply pervades signification and its very intelligibility. Ambiguity can be said to saturate the space of interiority between one and her (so-called) self in ways that disclose figuratively the interior monologue within when depicted as the relationship of thinking. It is then not vulgar to reflect upon the Grey Zone as the irreparable tension in thought thinking itself. This would make Hannah Arendt's work, *The Life of the Mind* (1978), an essential contribution to the formulation of the Grey Zone.

I use the Grey Zone to make reference to the instability of conceptions as symptoms rather than as facts to adjudicate, and so, as signs of the fundamental ambiguity of communication and of this terrain as a research opportunity. In this work I propose as usual that our routine vexatious engagement with the problem of irresolution in each and any shape must occur within the context of an interpretive landscape ruled by the need and desire for objectification and for reconciling such requirements in ways that are healthy, and where the normativity of any such standard continues to remind us of the remains that do and will remain in various iterated signs of intractable ambiguity. As our equipment for living, what we claim to know in the best sense must be measured by its capacity to heal ambiguity. Such a measure is complicated by the fact that the concern for subjectivity always must work within and against the technical horizon of social engineering and of the sciences, which typically imply that the message communicated is self-evident and can only be compromised by technical obstacles, and that communication is over once the message is received, then becoming the user's problem.[1]

My guiding question paraphrases Lenin's famous query "what is to be done?" by asking how a reflective subject is supposed to *be* under the desperate conditions of a normal life and the fundamental ambiguity it has to raise in the shape of many and diverse enigmatic conundrums, and especially at periods of life when such a question challenges us to dwell upon our expectation of learning from the past and influencing the future. The relation of the subject to such a challenge and the capacities for a healthy jouissance under such conditions is the object of this study.

Death as a Social Phenomenon

An example of the Grey Zone in this book is the relationship to dying and death as a situation of social action, whether attuned or not, as a living experience. I begin by reflecting upon the fear of death as part of a collective representation that seems to be animated by the unsettling character of our existence in time (the unknown future) and in space (the unstable referent) but might be engaged more reflectively as anxiety produced by materialist conceptions of the social actor and of the environment of action, including the body and the discourse that is in part created by concerns for how it is reciprocally involved in mindedness. Thus, if dying can be ruled by the thought of death as a matter considered in life, and so, as part of life, death itself tends to remind us of the inaccessibility of its notion (of its meaning as anything but a brute fact) as a sign of the limits of constructive activity.

My topic in this work is the collective engagement with death and the usage I examine includes many examples of the ways in which the fact of death is encountered in life. This leads me to navigate a discourse on death—on its place in life—as a way of addressing the relationship as a social phenomenon. In the idiom of sociology, death is a social fact, a relationship to which we orient and that must appear for us in the shape of this discourse and its conventions. These conventions surrounding death frame and structure such a relationship both as limit and incentive for the work of analysis.

The main focus on death through the ages has not been directed to supplying a cure for it (despite occasional fantasies) but in relieving the fear of it, first by asking whether or not we should fear it, and then after deciding one way or another, constructing for ourselves some kind of medicine, usually to relieve the fear, or if not, to justify those kinds of accounts that counsel fearlessness. The undercurrent here is that the apparent anonymity of the enterprise must connect in some way to the intimacy of death for one who contemplates such as me, the self-absorption of this event always confirming that the fear being studied must touch the inquiring one who proposes to study it. The inevitability of death suggests not simply the unalterability of the limit but through the types of evasions it brings to view, an often comedic spectacle of any solution claiming to be empirical or logical, showing in its way how ludicrous it is to argue for and against death on behavioral grounds, or by making arguments as Anglo-American philosophers often try in order to overcome their anxieties. As the Greeks suggested through the example of Hesiod the shepherd, each of these approaches can be seen as whistling in the dark. So the discourse on death reveals a fear that is quite complex in its way as a social phenomenon oriented to problem-solving that includes the comedic gestures of philosophers, the tragic spell of laments, refrains, odes in grieving, and the variety of means of expressing the fear in ways intending to deliver palliative care in the form of healing. Besides all of these, the discourse summons up the prospect of art and its endeavors as part of the need and desire to relieve the gloom and doom that death must raise as its residue.

The force of art in this discourse has been described by Matthew von Unwerth as illustrated in the exchange between Rilke and Freud where they each try to situate the poet and, implicitly art in relation to transience, asking in their different ways how it is possible to live in the face of death. In formulating the bell from Schiller's poem, according to von Unwerth, Freud treats necessity (*ananke*) as

> the single force that our collective ingenuity cannot dominate. It is the emblem of all human striving against the inevitable decline and extinction we face, as an individual and as a race … the bell stands in a word for poetry, by which an artist shoulders the burden of creation and the even heavier knowledge of the transient fate of that creation—and yet takes it up anyway.
>
> (von Unwerth 2005, 146)

We see here that healing is topicalized through the hesitation that Freud presumably expresses for von Unwerth in his words that the artist "yet takes it up anyway."

Jouissance of the dying body is "taken up," treated as its own necessity in a way that Freud accepts as equipment for living, necessary for an art of healing but in a way that Rilke finds astonishing.

> Murderers are easy
> to understand. But this: that one can contain
> death, the whole of death, even before
> life has begun, can hold it to one's heart
> gently, and not refuse to go on living,
> is inexpressible.
>
> (Rilke's Fourth Elegy, quoted in von Unwerth 2005, 152)

That the dying body keeps at life is harder to understand than the motive of murder and, unlike this terrain, seems inexpressible. Life is harder to understand than crime. Here we squarely face the motive for life, to live, that all accept without question and that Rilke finds enigmatic. The discourse on death is a discourse that can exhibit the healing powers of art as a collection of ways of engaging finitude, but only as an art guided by reflective thought or philosophy at its best. The discourse on death begins to reveal life to us as somewhat miraculous, giving substance to Baudrillard's inversion of Heidegger's question by converting it as "why is there nothing rather than something?" Why do we keep at life under these conditions? This question invites us to investigate the accounts and representations we offer for continuing to live with vitality.

Since I take up many of these themes in one way or another in this work, the topic is not so much death but its narrative and aesthetic force as a catalyst in the life of the dying body as equipment for living in order to deal with the fear of death as a problem in this situation. In the idiom of sociology, death is a situation of action addressed to "solving" the problem of its fear; in the therapeutic idiom of the best of medicine, it makes reference to a situation ruled by the need to develop a way of healing the fear. Imagining another idiom, Lacan might ask if a jouissance of the dying body is possible and, if so, how it might it be administered.

Death and the Grey Zone

In a way similar to all distinctions and distinguishing, the notion of the Grey Zone is not immediately accessible but comes to view on occasions when ambiguity appears sufficiently unsettling to be anxiety provoking, an occasion typically made compelling for the many by their encounter with death, but as Jonathan Strauss (2000) argues, that can become transparent in any impasse marked by figurative language in the "negativity" it assumes. Death tends to bring us together to face the Grey Zone and the implications it releases, a fact that we easily recognize at the moment of disasters, emergencies, or critical life-threatening events and, of course, at funerals and on occasions of grieving or stewardship for chronic disease and illness. This suggests that if the Grey Zone is a constant source of tension capable of becoming manifest throughout life, it typically needs to be displaced in energetic activity, often repressed, perhaps denied, disavowed, foreclosed, and reinstated in different shapes. Yet, the so-called denial of death is not unhappy if handled with an art that aims to resist absorption by a phobic preoccupation with its "fact" that interrupts our life and commitment to any present. In this respect, what the Greeks called the aporia, as that moment when stable relations to speech and action are unsettled by questioning, can also be marked as the critical moment when the tie to life and the point of its actions of distinguishing is desanctified in the recognition of its immanent loss:

> One knows that what is coming is death. This death is not one of an array of possibilities one reaches out for and takes hold of; it is for the dying one the end of all possibilities, impossibility itself. All of the experience and skills one has acquired are powerless to deal with it… . There is nothing to do but suffer and wait for death… . The present stretches out without passing, without going anywhere.
>
> (Lingis 2000, 110)

Although death, as such an awareness, seems to illustrate best the relationship to bare life within life itself that Agamben ([1982] 2006, 17) dramatizes in the recognition that "the limit of language always falls within language itself," derived from Wittgenstein among others (from Parmenides through Hegel and beyond), Strauss (2000) argues against this paradigmatic use of death as limited in the way an ontological view as this must assume its ground in the Grey Zone as another manifestation, and so, as a symptom rather than cause of the trauma of ambiguity.

Thus, Strauss discusses ways in which what he calls an "ontological" view of death allows us to neutralize it by seeing it as a mark of meaninglessness and limit that actually prevents us from appreciating the specificity of death and its connection to the particular character of the loss. That is, the singularity of the relationship to death as my death and only mine even as it happens to everyone (its form in the idiom of Plato) risks being denied when reiterated in abstractions that use it to personify an engagement with meaninglessness, because the particularity of death as a social relationship, though depicted in endless detail, can be foreclosed in such theorizing. What is particular to death is not simply its raising the problem of limit and meaning but how the loss of an intimate history that it dramatizes is integrated in life in any present. What Strauss calls the "ontological" view of death makes reference to the notion of the relativism of death as a condition that all must suffer, and so, a condition that all submit to equally as a common exigency to be endured, in contrast to the particular fact of death experienced by and for the subject who encounters it as a singular and absolute loss that is specific and unique. Instead of arguing for either or one of these views we consider them as positions in a discourse on death and a source of tension in relationships to death. Death then has two registers that interact to create a tension for the subject between its relativistic status as something that happens to all as if an anonymous condition of life (which Strauss calls ontological) and an intimate experience as something happening to the subject in a unique way that reveals a particular kind of dispossession and loss felt in a singular way. These two registers of death, that it happens to all as shared and to each uniquely and irrevocably singular, is a focus and ethical collision that we will pursue throughout.

For example, death summons to mind for me my engagement with myself as irrevocably mine even though such an experience might be shared by all and "relative" in that sense, absolutely mine as the perpetual lost object, the object in a state of dispossession, myself as once possessed and to be lost. Here, the self is persistently posed as a question—was I here and, if so, what does it matter to me now and eternally? Did I imagine being here and what does it mean or is it the work of a deceiving God that tricked me into accepting this illusion? Indeed, one of the problems of extreme action is that it might always be a reply to the absence of such signs, a reply to the silence it imagines as indications of a commentary on life well spent or abused. In this way death can always invite us to do more with what we are and with what we have, to intervene in ways that are innovative in relation to this discourse that we inherit.

The problem arising from having to care for death, whether of our own or of the other(s), might then motivate us to reexamine the conditions of a vital life and of a commitment to vitality as something that we always need to nurture in the face of empirical conditions. This suggests care itself as another such condition as Heidegger noted long ago, where care for inescapable conditions becomes just as inescapable as part of our human condition. The point of such vitality then needs to be rethought under the auspices of the cliché that everyone dies alone and that no one can die for another. This remains true even while people live together or with others, and so, always invites us to ask how such separation and togetherness can be said to interact and what the best stories for representing such interrelations might be for us. Any story, as our equipment for living, would need to engage the question here of best practices, how we might be said to live together *and* to die alone. One of my purposes in this work is to imagine and plot such a course of action or healing for a subject (the ideal speaker) I conceive as needing and desiring to embody the "as-if" of commitment to any present. Thus, one of my objectives is to formulate the dying life as a course of social action that materializes as one way of administering jouissance. Of course many can be seen to prepare for this, to rehearse in a way, by deciding to live alone. How we all engage and negotiate this impasse is the focus of our study. But then again, do we not all live alone with our archive of impressions even in the midst of others?

This contrast between the anonymity and intimacy of death has been developed in different ways, for example, by Robert Pogue Harrison (2003) in his focus upon loss and grief (developed from Vico and formulated as a contrast to Heidegger), in Judith Butler's (2000) distinction between the particularity of Antigone's appeal to family and burial as intimate testimony rather than as simply ontological as she attributes to the readings of the play by Hegel and Lacan, and in Dumm's (2008) work on *Loneliness as a Way of Life*. In these views, death promises a recovery of the connections between intimacy and solidarity in human existence as a means of explicating the cliché that no one can die for another. Lacan, for example, does persistently dramatize this difference in his contrast between death as seen by oneself and death treated as objectified from the perspective of Other, suggesting in this way that for anyone death is divided both as absolute and as other, as only belonging to me (intimate), and yet as belonging to everyone (anonymous). So while it is true that everyone and anyone dies alone and is equal in that sense, and that everyone and anyone might seem to experience this common destination in the same way with trepidation perhaps, they (we) all seem to confront our death as singular in relation to "content" that in its way seems unique to its subject. Again, it is Franz Rosenzweig who is reputed to exemplify the recognition of this point of tension in death and not in any other signifier, its singular character that dramatizes this relationship between the absolutism of my death and the relativism of death for Other as summarized by Blond: "The uniqueness of human finitude cannot be encompassed by any universal framework, exemplified in the particularity of one's own death. Because death is an event related to the particular, experiential individual, it cannot be understood in terms of a general characteristic. In this way, the defiance of death individuates a human being" (Blond 2010, 43).

Conclusion

Is this tendency to both absolutize and relativize ourselves not the primordial illumination of the Grey Zone, of the (dis)connection of intimacy and anonymity, ideal and material, as if comingling in the lived experience we all call our self? If everyone truly dies alone, the life world of the dying body can be infected by this apprehension, allowing this sense of solitude to rule the subject, and thereby posing for the life of dying the task and challenge of breaking the habit of this emphasis on solitude as isolation.[2]

Notes

1 For those familiar with Lacan's idiom, the Grey Zone is a sociological translation of object a and its materialization in different ways and guises and is intelligible as the working-out of jouissance in everyday life, accessible to us and to theorizing as the panorama of non-dialectical relations to the limit that we call symptoms and all such adaptations.

2 Anthony Lane (2014, 118) notes this in his postscript on the actor Philip Seymour Hoffman in treating his habit of solitude as a kind of addiction and a force in his creativity: "From early on, this was what we treasured in Hoffman: his will to break the habit of solitude—all the more so because we realize what a crushing addiction it can be."

References

Agamben, Giorgio. (1982) 2006. *Language and Death: The Place of Negativity*. Translated by Karen E. Pinkus and Michael Hardt. Minneapolis: University of Minnesota Press.

Arendt, Hannah. 1978. *The Life of the Mind*. Edited by Mary McCarthy. New York: Harcourt Brace Jovanovich.

Blond, Louis P. 2010. "Franz Rosenzweig: Homelessness in Time." *New German Critique* 111: 27–58.

Butler, Judith. 2000. *Antigone's Claim: Kinship Between Life and Death*. New York: Columbia University Press.

Dumm, Thomas. 2008. *Loneliness as a Way of Life*. Cambridge, MA: Harvard University Press.

Harrison, Robert Pogue. 2003. *The Dominion of the Dead*. Chicago: University of Chicago Press.

Lane, Anthony. 2014. "Remembering Phillip Seymour Hoffman." *The New Yorker*, February 17 and 24, 116–119.

Lingis, Alphonso. 2000. "To Die With Others." *Diacritics* 30 (3): 106–113.

Serres, Michel. (1991) 1997. *The Troubadour of Knowledge*. Translated by Sheila Faria Glaser with William Paulson. Ann Arbor: University of Michigan Press.

Strauss, Jonathan. 2000. "Preface: The State of Death." *Diacritics* 30 (3): 3–11.

Von Unwerth, Matthew. 2005. *Freud's Requiem: Mourning, Memory, and the Invisible History of a Summer Walk*. New York: Riverhead Books.

2 Fear and Trembling

Introduction

I begin to lay out the parameters of the collective fascination with death as an "object" reflected in Kierkegaard's title that grips us as a riveting concern even if surreptitiously avoided. I want to trace both the inevitability of death and the fear it arouses as an aspect of the imaginary structure of materialism that posits it as an inescapable and unalterable condition framing what I think of as a problem-solving situation for the human subject. The chapters begin to lay out this interpretive terrain and the need and desire to address it in action as the fate of the social actor. Though this usage is common currency and part of the collective orthodoxy, it constitutes a necessary beginning in this work for analysis and research. One can say that analysis and research on death is one way of dealing with it, though not necessarily of avoiding it. If the inevitability of death can stimulate us to reflect upon our limits, this "contribution" risks being abstract and relatively anonymous in contrast to the traumatic confrontation with our intimate experience of dispossession that it arouses. Throughout I try to refocus Kenneth Burke's (1957) conception of our propensity to convert our handicaps into virtues that he locates in poetry as the task of converting our sense of annihilation into an engagement with the infinite perplexity of finitude without the aid of miraculous solutions.

My objective is to lay grounds for relating to fear and trembling as the unspoken undercurrent concealed in all social action, and so, as a necessity for hearing what seems unsaid and in acting upon self and other(s) strongly by managing in some way to avoid nihilism while treating everyone and anyone as innocent in relation to Being. The lived experience of the dying body is identified at this point as the need and desire to resist acting out in relation to the sorrow of finitude, to break the habit of solitude through an inclination to improvise experimentally with the jouissance of any present.

The Matter of Human Life: Ideal and Material

The primordial text on materialism attributed to Lucretius ([50 BCE] 1965) emphasizes the fundamental tension between happiness and society. Here, the happiness of people in the ideal society can only be based on a "reigning delusion" in which time is seen as eternal and space as permeable. In this deluded state, before humans are truly reflective, they can only treat the present moment as eternal because it is viewed as unchanging, just as the limits of their society are viewed as if "walls of the world" (Strauss 1953 on Lucretius, 112–114). Thus, for materialism, idealism is only happy because it lives in error, and commitment to the ideal is doomed to be false. According to this materialism, philosophy inspires humans to break through such insularity by recognizing that "society" (the social) is only a nominal creation of the totemic convention that ranks its part *as* the whole and its time *as* eternal. In breaking through the "walls of the world" we come to recognize the void (that we are "really" bodies, bits and pieces, fragments in space), flux (that irrational fluctuation and motion is the "real" law of the cosmos), and relativism (that we are not immune to coming-to-be and perishing, and that we are "really" ruled by perspective, by the time and space we *happen* to occupy). This "breakthrough" is the achievement of a truthful if unhappy recognition. Of course, in achieving this recognition, we also come to understand that the idols we had lived by and accepted on faith or trustingly (for example, religion) were delusions. Lucretius tells us that, at any present moment, our life is a struggle with the happy and deluded temptation of idealism. Being strong in the present requires the will to live with the unhappy truth that life is a hollow bubble and that we are condemned to be here today and gone tomorrow. It is interesting how this counsel echoes in Max Weber's ([1921–1922] 1947) modern advice to those who would turn their backs on reality that "the arms of the church are open" to you if you cannot endure these "stern and fateful times." We might recognize here the high testosterone level of materialism in all of its shapes.

The rhetoric of loss is interesting as a materialist preoccupation and appears in much research on the city. In this respect, Herbert Marcuse (1964) said of one version of classical hedonism that it was tempted to treat true interests as atrophied and repressed. In this way, Marcuse permits us to link much of Lucretius' notion of the lost happy state of deluded idealism to Kant's sense that the depth of any relation to the distinction (to the in-itself) invariably appears as lost (that is, as irretrievable in our present situation). It is said that idealism depends upon a situation favorable to it that is lost (the Greek city-state?) and, in this way, must be linked to history, contingency, and fluctuations as if its time is past. It is as if truth is so traumatic that it cures us of idealism (in the way Adorno thinks of the end of art after the Holocaust). In the idiom of Socrates, materialism shows a curious misology here, since the distrust in reason that it reveals appears to be based on the capacity of truth to terrify us into relinquishing any concern for the ideal (as in the cliché that says "welcome to real life," or in the parental admonition that expects children to lose their "ideals" as they mature). It is said that knowledge and happiness cannot coexist because any truth worth its name is reputed to suffer the fate of losing its innocence, and so, philosophy, as the preoccupation of grown-ups, is condemned to the gravity of an unhappy life (see the character of Callicles, who chides Socrates to grow up and escape his nursemaid whom he is accused of needing to wipe his nose, in Plato's *Gorgias*).

According to this view, since it was the state of ignorance that gave us comfort, truth can only coexist with unhappiness because this society is gone, never to be regained, and even if it could be miraculously recovered, living it would be a lie since it was founded on error. The truthful grasp of our society can only lead to unhappiness: "we live in an unwalled city, in an infinite universe in which nothing that man can love can be eternal" (Strauss 1953, 113). In Book 1 of his work, Lucretius ([50 BCE] 1965, I.ii.958–959) counsels us that it is not only the universe that is unbounded but that there is no limit to division, suggesting that any distinction masks the essential intermingling of bodies of matter that "fly about for ever unvanquished through the ages." That is, if distinction is the basis of any social order and its totemic principles, reflection can only be the fateful and unhappy recognition of the capricious intermingling of everything. If we all, including the materialist, live in society, and if society is founded on the conventions of classification and naming, then knowledge of society is knowledge of its errors, of living in error (living as if my part was the whole, living as if my time was eternal). Materialist doctrine seeks to cure us of the superstition of false humanism founded on an essentialist and utopian "reign of delusion." Therefore, if the social order keeps apart reflection and happiness, as if this separation is a condition of life, it could also show ethical collisions over this relationship and, perhaps, ways and means of navigating this abutment.

Materialism says that nothing remains eternal and everything is in movement, that is, life conceived as a body is in a constant state of dismemberment. Knowledge, whether idealism or rationalism, is viewed as defending itself from this true recognition with interpretations that can only mask the deadly movement of life. Under such conditions happiness is false (impossible), because it is simply innocent enthusiasm based upon ignorance of the truth, while yet truth cannot produce happiness because it knows that life is an illusion and must live in painful recognition of what it knows. Inner isolation is expressed both in the distractedness of innocent and ignorant enthusiasm and in the morbidity of the impotent skepticism that sees truly. What materialism knows is that the body takes no prisoners, leaving no space for ambiguity and its reflection. Everything is a false image that simply defers the true recognition that there is no "original" other than the deadly movement of corporeality. Yet, even in this way, what is lost or dead, in showing itself as an absence *that remains present to us as lost*, can only cast its uncanny spell on the present as an objective to be restored, pursued, or simply acknowledged in its way.

This oppressive equality that links us all by virtue of the death we must share seems to make our sense of difference, whether as individual or species, vainglorious, and so, laughable. Lucretius still remains the exemplary spokesman for this view:

> Finally, what great and evil desire for life forces us to such restless activity amid dangers of uncertain outcome? Truly a sure termination of life stands near at hand for mortals, nor can we avoid the meeting with death. Moreover, we spin about in the same place and are still present there, nor do we forge,

> by living, any new pleasures for ourselves. But while what we desire is absent, it seems superior to other things; when we have gained this, we seek for something else, and an unchanged thirst for life still holds us open-mouthed. Lastly, there is doubt what fortune time may bring, what may be sent to us by chance, what end is pressing upon us. By prolonging life we do not diminish by a hair the period of death, nor can we take anything away from it so that we may be dead less long. Finally, although by your living you bring to an end as many generations as you please, yet the death that awaits you will be none the less eternal; and he who made an end of life today will be dead no less long than he who died many months and years ago.
>
> (Lucretius [50 BCE] 1965, 113)

The ignorance or delusion derided by Lucretius as the belief in immortality for which there is no proof, or the frenzied preoccupation with death at which he sneers rather than analyzes, seems a superstition analogous to the maxim of Socratic ignorance. The life-sustaining stories of Socrates to his friends about the immortality of the soul, reflecting the drive to live inspired by human anxiety in the relation to the unknown that is evoked by death, intelligible as the desire to live forever in the face of knowing its impossibility, is much like the maxim of Socratic ignorance and its counsel to pursue knowledge, though one can never know more than their ignorance, that is, to pursue the desire to know in the face of its impossibility. We can think of this as a version of Lacan's drive, jouissance, the necessary and desirable desire for the impossible, and so as a death drive that insists to live.

If nothing lasts, going on can seem as ludicrous as the maxim of Socratic ignorance that honors the desire for knowledge in the face of its impossible realization. As Nietzsche affirms, the sense of the groundlessness of Being makes inaction appear necessary and action ludicrous. The coexistence of the desire for life and the knowledge of the inevitability of death stirs in the human soul in relation to the uncanny foreboding of disappearance in all that exists and in all that we hold dear. Thus, in reply to Lucretius, we could only point to him and to his image, to his circulation as a life force, and so, as real, as an aesthetic phenomenon. But then this is as accidental as the silence that might follow any other death in the fortuitous event of its lack of such influences or successors. That is, we might not be as lucky as Lucretius, or as talented! Here we are not simply saying that the relationship to death requires respite as a kind of escapism or denial but that the aesthetic character of existence seems to invite the self-understanding of mortality as the kind of justification that neither knowledge nor ethics can provide, and in the words of Rancière's reformulation of Kant's disengagement or notion of form, appears as a "double negation."

Finding our place or the center in a world marked by apparent infinitization shows the pain of truth that has to be reconciled. If the reconciliation is between truth and meaning, it seems more directly posed not around the issue of desire but in terms of what Lacan calls drive as a kind of insistence almost corporeal, asking how to be resolute and life-affirming in the present while knowing the truth of the groundlessness of being. Thus, we can invert Spinoza's axiom that we pursue the worst knowing the best by affirming that we pursue the best (life) knowing the worst (death). The pain of this work involves concealing what is true as a kind of self-deception that is yet true to the necessity of life. It is as if life lies against truth, that embracing the present is a lie, while standing "frankly" for the truth is deadly.

Matter, Imagination, Malleability

Note the time-honored Aristotelian conception of matter as both primary material (determination, being determined in the way of a statue), and determinability (potential, capacity of indetermination to be determined in the way marble is determined as the statue).

> A material reality is what it is in such a way that it bears in itself the possibility of simply not being what it is ... any determination one considers of itself implies inadequacy. It would not make sense, of course, to posit this inadequacy apart from the determination.
>
> (Luytun [1963] 1965, 108)

The thing made bears as its nature the capacity to be otherwise in the way the statue reflects the potential of malleable marble to assume many shapes, thus marking the statue as one of these shapes, and so, as "deficient" in the way Other stands to the Same as one of its parts and as inadequate in this sense. That is, the otherness of marble is this capacity for diversification. Yet, if partiality is deficient in relation to a whole (the statue in relation to marble), the whole seems deficient in so far as it needs the parts to give it life (insofar as marble remains indeterminate without the determination given by the statue). The malleability of matter shows this kind of neediness as unending circulation, mutation, marking the Same as requiring determination. As sheer potential, the Same would be ethereal or an empty abstraction without the determination of statue (and many other of its shapes) to be seen as what it is in ways that make these shapes intrinsic rather than external to matter as what it is. This means that the indeterminacy is seen through what it determines as what is indeterminacy. This needful relation is reversed in the case of the statue for without matter, it could not be the statue it is, this marble being that communalizes each and all of the shapes. More, the fact that a convention can be otherwise (McHugh 1970) can be expressed in this Aristotelian lingo as inadequacy or deficiency, or today through the figure of the signifier that is determined and can be otherwise (its potentiality or signification cannot be shown apart from its determination as what it is). This reiterates the relation of Same to Other as indetermination to a determinate thing, or in Hegel as the infinite to the finite.

> And so one may conclude that there is no absurdity in admitting a real pure indetermination, provided that one does not posit it as a reality existing in itself, but rather as a constitutive deficiency of the given material thing.
>
> (Luytun [1963] 1965, 108)

Peter McHugh and I (1984) treated this relation (in Hegel) between discourse and the absolute as a figure for the tension noted here, saying that just as discourse "needs" the absolute (in the way the statue needs the marble), so the absolute needs the discourse (in the way the marble needs the statue). Note also though that the statue's need for the marble is not incomparable for it could be made by other material, and the marble also can find itself in fountains, kitchen tops, and many kinds of things. So all of these relations can be otherwise, can take other shape(s), but the absolute is special in a way that the determinations are not by virtue of determination per se. What is other than determination is indistinction, which we must determine as such. We cannot escape from having to distinguish, making what is absolute not the distinction per se, but the relation of a distinction to indistinction. This is to say that the relation of indistinction to distinction is absolute for the living and if the dead were imaginable they would have to be distinguished as such: the distinction that can be otherwise shows us in its appearance the relationship that is absolute and cannot be otherwise.

Indifferent to Lacan at this time, what Peter McHugh and I did was translate this vision of materiality and its malleability into an image of speech and its auspices or grounds as a relationship that Lacan had envisioned between Other and the signifier, through the *physis* of signification. This was adumbrated in Hegel's conception of the relation of the finite to infinity and the twin errors of reducing the infinite to the finite (and the either/or) and of separating the infinite from the finite (from the either/or), instead of developing their relationship.

Thus, what the Aristotelian image of matter calls pure indetermination is the Grey Zone, understood not as a tangible material thing, but also not intelligible apart from determinate things, that is, as a relationship between the indeterminate and determination that exists and is visible only through the appearances disclosed in determinate things such as distinctions. This relationship is pursued by thinking of indetermination as inadequate by virtue of its needing to be given shape as a determinate thing through determination (in the way Other needs signification).

Conclusion

The Grey Zone is not a concrete reality existing in and of itself but "it is a deficiency," that is, it indicates the possibility of this thing's becoming another thing ad infinitum. The "deficiency" can be read as a mark of infinity that is deficient or inadequate only in the sense of exceeding determination in ways that can only be revealed through determination. As with marble and the statue, we could be fooled if we thought that the matter of humans could never be otherwise, and so, if we identified our conventions of determining humanity as absolute. Figures such as inadequacy and deficiency must include our representations as such in ways that make the Grey Zone inescapable. In Hegel, the infinite is not apart from the finite (the indeterminate is not apart from the determinate thing), and neither is the infinite reducible to the finite, but there is a needful relation of each to the other. The ways we think about life and death and our various boundaries and limits could be otherwise (they are deficient or inadequate in this sense), but we only approach any matters through such distinctions, showing how what is absolute and cannot be otherwise is distinguishing as a relationship. We might even say that life needs distinguishing.

That the statue of a lion can be otherwise does not mean that it might have been made as a frog or a rabbit (true enough) but that its being made as a lion, as what it is, is deficient in terms of other ways of being true to the notion of a lion, and so, invariably falls short of such a notion, of being true to itself. Thus, the mix of infinite to finite lies not in the relation of the statue of the lion to other types of things but of the statue to itself. The lion as statue seems deficient or inadequate not simply because it is malleable and can or could have been made as a frog but for the reason that its lacking life, as a statue copying an animal, is always problematic. This identifies the "hole" in the symbolic order. The statue is like the dead letter that drives life. What is ambiguous revolves around the question of whether this is done well or poorly, and the "inadequacy" or "deficiency" here resides in the impossibility of an answer. This question always raised creates our everlasting fascination with animation as more than the malleability of the statue but with respect to life, death, the uncanny, Pygmalion, and the family of such effects. The deficiency of a good statue resides not in failing to be everything thinkable but in its being unable to solve the question of its relation to life for us, being deficient in that sense, and yet productive at the same time. Note that if what deficient matter produces is our sense of infinite perplexity, this applies to us as well insofar as our sharing such materiality makes it difficult to treat our self or the other as anything but a statue. Figuring out this relationship means that we always have work to do.

When the idea of deficiency is conceived not as an error resulting from our "failure" to be everything possible in the way being a lion is one thing but not everything, not the whole, being everything else is an impossibility rather than a failure; but being the best we can be as a lion is a different kind of limitation. That the human is not a God is not a deficiency or an error whereas a human's inability to be as good as a human can be might be inescapable and inevitable in the way of a limit rather than a lack, something like an incapacity. Both of these ideas of impossibility and incapacity make reference to the notion of limit intrinsic to being rather than to lack or failure.

References

Blum, Alan and Peter McHugh. 1984. *Self-Reflection in the Arts and Sciences*. Atlantic Highlands, NJ: Humanities Press.

Burke, Kenneth. 1957. *The Philosophy of Literary Form: Studies in Symbolic Action.* Berkeley, CA: University of California Press.

Lucretius. (50 BCE) 1965. *On Nature*. Translated by R.M. Geer. Indianapolis: Bobbs-Merrill.

Luytun, Norman. (1963) 1965. "Matters as Potency." In *The Concept of Matter in Greek and Medieval Philosophy*, 102–113. Notre Dame, IN: University of Notre Dame Press.

Marcuse, Herbert. 1964. *One-Dimensional Man: Studies in the Ideology of Advanced Industrial Society*. Boston: Beacon Press.

McHugh, Peter. 1970. "A Common-Sense Perception of Deviance." In *Recent Sociology No. 2: Patterns of Communication,* edited by H.P. Dreitzel, 151–180. New York: Macmillan.

Strauss, Leo. 1953. *Natural Right and History*. Chicago: University of Chicago Press.

3 The Collective Fantasizes Death—the Imaginary at the end of its Tether

Introduction

If the cryptic remark attributed to Lacan that birth is an event of distress appears to counteract the celebratory view of birth, it is not because of the painful labor of childbearing, but because of the promise implicit in the induction of any and every human into the symbolic order with respect to the travail of ambiguity that will need to be engaged and developed in relation to the condition of mortality. Following Arendt, Kieran Bonner (1998) analyzes such awaiting as interruption. What is inherited by every human is the need to meditate upon the condition of mediation, which seems impossible because we cannot imagine the absence of mediation, while yet speaking it as such seems to suggest that this impossibility is possible. Thus, the idea of birth as an event of distress is imagined as the moment when the in-between character of life as awaiting becomes poignant, suggesting that the best of reflection must grasp the irony of this mix of living and dying as jouissance, the insistence of the drive of life (narcissism, self-preservation) for the one who must suffer the pain of this distress wordlessly.

Jean Laplanche ([1970] 1976) discusses a paper of Freud's that concludes "the bearing of life is the first duty of every human being," translating Freud's use of the maxim "if you seek peace prepare for war" into "if you would endure life prepare for death," that is, your death! Laplanche continues:

> In the unconscious, death would always be the death of the other, a destruction or loss we provoke, and we would accede to some intuition of our own mortality only through an ambivalent identification with a loved person. If a certain ethic in relation to death might be evolved from the Freudian attitude, it would be in the sense of a distrust concerning every form of enthusiasm, be it that of *amor fati*, and of a lucidity that does not hide the irreducible meshing of my death with that of the other.
>
> (8)

Despite the ethical overtones to which Laplanche points, Freud's notion of the denial of death introduces a tension between the ethical and the aesthetic organized around the ambiguity of enthusiasm itself as a signifier, two-sided in its need to distance itself from the mindless and self-absorbed embrace of existence (that forgets the connection between the death of the other and of oneself) and yet needs to accept with enthusiasm rather than resignation the "bearing of life."

> My death, an unreal question: as long as I am, it is not, and if it is, I am not any more. This we've known since antiquity, and such knowledge has never been any use to anyone for anything and is for everyone who approaches death only a tasteless joke. It is true. It is false. It is wisdom and folly. In fact, every subjective utterance about one's own death contains a logical problem. I am not. Doesn't this "I am" exclude the "not?" Not insofar as my utterance lets me both take myself out of myself and view my nonbeing or not-being-here as an objective fact, i.e., from the perspective of the survivor. Yes, the "I am" does not allow a "not" if I stay within myself and understand my ego as that which alone can have sense for me: as something being here… . The event of my death, the fact of my death, which in spite of all its logical problems concerns me more than all others and everything else, is only comprehensible for the survivors and only by them to be integrated into the course of affairs.
>
> (Améry [1968] 1994, 107–108)

But then Améry committed suicide. Can we dare rethink the question of the tension in the idea of life and death as functional and no more, and of productivity and reproduction as illusory, the idea of the living death, bare life, your money or your life, the death drive, and the assorted moves in the symbolic order and imaginative structure of life and death? In this way, the traditional forms—philosophy, art, and politics—could appear as if light-hearted replies to such a grave matter, or as grave responses to a light-hearted matter. This is one question we consider: how do humans reply to the gravity of death, by imitating such gravity or in comic ways? In *Waiting for Godot* Beckett used waiting to depict existence and not death, showing existence (not being) as commensurate with anticipation and expectation, although commentators have tended to treat his view of existence as living death (where it might be more accurate to say that existence is neither life nor death but the lived experience of the dying body).

Can a person live in a way that expresses fear and trembling, without desperation or severity, but in a light-hearted manner that inflects the obscurity of this intermediate position between birth and death, a position that neither simply endures waiting nor devotes itself to movement, but moves while waiting and waits in the midst of movement? Such a pose might need to engage a subject imaginatively who occupies this space whether masterfully or ludicrously, always keeping its eye on the space itself rather than the content, the space as medium and message.

> [E]very individual life between birth and death can eventually be told as a story with beginning and end. The perplexity is that in any series of events that together form a story with a unique meaning we can at best isolate the agent who set the whole process into motion; and although this agent

> frequently remains the subject, the "hero" of the story, we can never point unequivocally to him as the author of its eventual outcome.
>
> (Arendt 1958, 184–185)

If what birth and death have in common is such a frame, being the first and last chapters of a story, the story itself does not seem to have a beginning or an end. This is because the subject, the "who" or author of the outcome of the story (and indeed the story of the outcome) is fundamentally ambiguous and cannot be identified "unequivocally," making it forever revisable according to the image's decomposition as it circulates in life. It is necessary for we who live to suffer in anticipation that the subject of our story will perhaps be misrecognized and certainly will circulate in an interpretive landscape that can only be oriented to as unknown.

What is unknown is the story that will be told of us, and it is this one thing that we know. Is this a view of the possibility of impossibility that animates Heidegger's reflections on death and Derrida's reformulation that it is impossible to know the story but that this impossibility as such belongs to us?

What is sacrificed is the ideal of hermeneutic finality that imparts to the story its sense of phallic final judgment, for in contrast, its dream of a perpetuity of dialogue. The story of any life is much like a dream that sacrifices its conception of a conclusion and of conclusiveness to the image of its circulation in a future conversation that will unmake and remake its text. This notion of the life as a dream also applies to the method of seeing the meaning of any practice by seeking to recover its voice and implicitly its dream, in any situation. In this way, for any practice the realization of desire, whether mine or the other, is always unknown as an opener, inspired by the dream of its realization of desire in the future, at a site for the engagement with meaning. This relation of the recovery of voice to the maintenance of community is not fundamentalist but an image of a perpetual place where meaning will be discussed and discussion will continue to be supported. When tyranny uses force to extinguish this imagined line and legacy of perpetual support, desolation can condemn the subject to a present detached from future.

This tells us that though the individual is enclosed between birth and death, beginning and ending with such definitiveness, that the story of the individual can be recreated in a way that is unending, born again in many ways, and ending over and again: that even with the death, the existence of the story does not seem to conclude. This inconclusiveness belongs to the story as its structure of fortuitous possibilities. And will the "content" of this story not express the tension at the heart of its status as an image between its being a likeness of a life and the simulacrum that reinvents this life as such? Yet, we should not be too confident about the unending story because, as Hegel warned, the barbarians can come or the ice age can materialize again, that is, because jouissance is absolute for us but relative for Other.

Wishful Thinking

> There is a substantial difference … between the philosophical truth of death and the philological certainty of the dead. Before it became the ultimate, unrepresentable possibility of my own impossibility of being—indeed, before it became exclusively mine—death wore the mask of the dead. Heidegger insists that *Dasein* cannot relate to its own death by way of the death of others (he calls death "non relational"), yet, this is as philosophically inadequate as his reduction of the corpse to mere presence-at-hand.
>
> (Pogue Harrison 2003, 93–94)

Yet, opposing dying to death, or relational to non-relational views of death in this way simply reverses Heidegger's procedure into more of the Same, for this makes reference to a trajectory in the collective representation, the trajectory that Lacan depicted between absolutism to and for the individual and relativism in relation to Other, showing the two-sided nature of the usage on death, intimate and external, as irreconcilable. Perhaps, in this case, what we wish for is that death be indivisible, and that we might overcome such ambiguity to gain a degree of assurance. What Heidegger misses is that in the death of the intimate some part of us dies insofar as our intimacy shares something that is perishable, reminding me that with his or her death, I am a custodian of the archive that will also expire with my death. What is between us and only us will die.

To wish for a condition to be overcome in the case of death is not to wish it away, but to wish for the end of the separation between life and death, as in the hope that life would be able to comprehend death in thought. In this sense wishful thinking is the wish to end a line of thought, the wish that a kind of thought would end, would die. Heidegger's lively thought is riddled with death in this sense: he wishes feverishly for the death of repulsive thought, of thought that doesn't think Being. Heidegger shows here the difference between death and extermination: although he calls everyone to the mission of thinking Being, and so, thinking life and death, he needs to exterminate those who do not heed the call. Wishful thinking wishes to exterminate bad conditions, conditions that obstruct purity, rather than analyze the thought that grounds such bad conditions as reasonable and good. For example, Heidegger ([1935] 1959, 185–186) wants language to be eventful, a "happening," rather than mere "chatter," and eventful speaking must engage the difference between Being and non-Being. But then language is immersed in "chatter," the chatter of the unconscious and its imaginary hold upon the speaker through resistance, the transference, and the force of narcissism, in ways that make chatter the symptom to be taken up by reflective thought, thought that seeks to analyze chatter rather than purge it, and to redeem chatterers rather than to exterminate them. Heidegger frequently says of genuine thought that it is limited to its horizon because "no one can jump over his shadow" (199), but to purge chatter and liquidate the chatterer is to try to jump over our shadow: when Heidegger calls *aletheia* the "struggle against … distortion and perversion" (192), he expurgates the phenomenon itself, the unconscious and its imaginary ruses of distorting and perverting as the very matter to be engaged and analyzed.

If talk about death could never be adequately formulated as ignorance, because there is no standard of knowledge against which its deficiency might be measured, the distinction between good and bad talk about death needs to be drawn elsewhere. Could we hazard in advance that good talk about death might, curiously enough, arouse our attachment to life? Pogue Harrison is right but diagnostically undeveloped here, for Heidegger's notion of a relationship to death that resists the fantastic effort to jump over its own shadow imagines it as the fate of dying at the hands of chatter, of being infected by the disease perpetuated by those others. The living death: death by transference, being determined by what we oppose, means that we see ourselves mirrored in the other for whom we bear such contempt, and that we begin to gather together vitality as we achieve separation that immunizes us. Here, what kills us is René Girard's ([1972] 1977) sacrificial crisis. Heidegger's reluctance to learn from the dead or from the death of others reflects this aversion to being influenced by the language of the living with respect to grief and loss, from the repetitive and formulaic chatter of life about the dead. (But then again Heidegger's readings of the past confirm how he does learn from the dead, if they are immune from his identification of chatter). For example, we can learn from the fragility of grief what is in store for us:

For in this world of ours where everything withers, everything perishes, there is a thing that decays, that crumbles into dust even more completely, leaving behind still fewer traces of itself, than beauty: namely grief. (Proust [1927] 2003, 7)

Here, wishful thinking might wish that grief and its preoccupation could last forever. Wishful thinking then can be understood as the desire for language to be other than it is, or in Heidegger's terms, to be a "happening," or eventful and not chatter. But if language always begins as chatter, or is unformed, empty, in need of development and resistance, it is as if Heidegger's wish is for any beginning to be an end, and so, in this case of death, that it is always engaged as itself eventful or a happening. In other words, it seems as if Heidegger wishes that speech about anything not be contaminated by the profanity of what is inessential in ways that desire to respect form on the one hand, the eventfulness of death as such, per se, but on the other hand can only cut off his theorizing of death from access to its imaginary character because such resonances must be treated by him as external. Here, Heidegger simplifies his own creation of *dasein* by excluding from this subject any depth or resonance greater than "anxiety." In other words, it is as if the imaginary relationship of *dasein* to being-there is treated with contempt. That is, Heidegger uses "anxiety" as an alibi to enable him not only to forget that *dasein* has an unconscious but to forget that he forgets. Heidegger just misses the point that his talk of death itself has to begin as chatter.

Stories

Lacan's ([1959–1960] 1992, 232) use of the figure of Oedipus as a placeholder for Anyman marks the conception of death suffered in Greek tragedy.

> Oedipus at Colonus … lives a life which is dead, which is that death which is precisely there under life. That is also where Freud's text leads us, where he tells us—don't believe that life is an exhalting goddess who has arisen to culminate in that most beautiful of forms, that there is the slightest power of achievement and progress in life. Life is a blister, a mould, characterized—as others besides Freud have written—by nothing beyond its aptitude for death. That is what life is—a detour, a dogged detour, in itself transitory and precarious, and deprived of any significance. Why, in that of its manifestations called man, does something happen, which insists throughout this life, which is called a meaning? We call it human but are we so sure? Is this meaning as human as all that?

If as Lacan suggests, this "happening" of meaning, its eventfulness and performance, insists itself upon the blister and mould of life, the "dogged detour" that can only be transitory and precarious and devoid of any significance, and if Lacan like any of us must write on and represent himself and his life as mattering, what seems most insistent is this desire, this aesthetic drive or need to perform at life, which his words both deny and reveal, the two-sidedness coexisting in the speech.

Yet for Oedipus, suffering the fluctuations of fortuna, the painful ambiguity of death must be linked to the unknown and to the question of immortality through the way in which reputation is in the hands of others. Although it seems as if such a fate applies only to the once great or famous men of action, and to the reversal of fortune that even their great deeds could not control, the idea of repute points to the fragility of the "object" that is "human," the destiny of which only dramatized in its reduction to a thing, to desublimation, disclosing how any object (any distinction, person) conceived in such a way is nothing unless perpetuated as something, is essentially in between nothing and something, the mortal object whose destiny lies in the hands of others and in the power of influences only discernible after as seeming to be integral to what it was before.

In contrast to the stories reflected in tragedy, Weber's ([1905] 1930) portrayal of the inner isolation (Blum 2003, 212) of Calvinist capitalism deprived of any reassurance for salvation can only produce the sense of life as requiring the gamble of work, of continuing to invest the normative with blind fervor in the expectation that methodical absorption in life is the only antidote to the caprice of fortuna.

> Human actions were deprived of all value. Something new arose: an empty world… . There was no answer to this except perhaps in the morality of ordinary people—"honesty in small things," "upright living"—which developed at this time… . For those who looked deeper saw the scene of their existence as a rubbish heap of partial, inauthentic actions. Life itself protested against this… . It is overcome by deep horror at the idea that the whole of existence might proceed in such a way. The idea of death fills it with profound terror. Mourning is the state of mind in which feeling revives the empty world in the form of a mask, and derives an enigmatic satisfaction in contemplating it.
>
> (Benjamin [1925] 1998, 138–139)

If Greek tragedy, Protestant asceticism, and melancholia each in their own way connect death to the limits of desire and the inability of Other to reply, to answer, then life can only be formulated as that which needs and desires to continue in the absence of such justification.

> Hamlet, the first wholly self-aware and despondently self-reflecting individual, experienced his essence as something absolutely transitory. In him the absolute experience of the individual as the self, and the experience of its absolute transience coincided. By contrast, it is probably the case today that, because the individual actually no longer exists, death has become something wholly incommensurable, the annihilation of a nothing. He who dies realizes he has been cheated of everything. And that is why death is so unbearable.
>
> (Adorno [1998] 2000, 136)

But as an example of the limit of such a gloss, note Freud ([1917] 1957, 255–257) on Hamlet and the tension between such truthfulness and sanity:

> He also seems to us justified in certain other self-accusations; it is merely that he has a keener eye for the truth than other people who are not melancholic. When in his heightened self-criticism he describes himself as petty, egoistic, dishonest, lacking in independence, one whose sole aim has been to hide the weaknesses of his whole nature, it may be, as far as we know, that he has come pretty near to understanding himself; we only wonder why a man has to be ill before he can be accessible to a truth of this kind. For there can be no doubt if anyone holds and expresses to others an opinion of himself such as this (an opinion which Hamlet held both of himself and of everyone else), he is ill, whether he is speaking the truth or whether he is being more or less unfair to himself… . Feelings of shame in front of other people … are lacking in the melancholic… . One might emphasize the presence in him of an almost opposite trait of insistent communicativeness which finds satisfaction in self-exposure… . The essential thing therefore, is not whether the melancholic's distressing self-denigration is correct… . The point must rather be that he is giving a correct description of his psychological situation. He has lost his self-respect and must have good reason for this.

Science fervently seeks a story that will allow its practitioners to avoid facing up to death, choosing to think about it as an example of the progressive march of paradigms, of increasing information, that will somehow "just around the corner" dissolve the problem, fascinated by the idea that death is another technical problem no different in kind from others, much like a disease that might be cured at some point.

But science often refuses to relinquish death to nature, especially in the guise of cryonics and the hope that future research will reveal secrets that might enable us to live, providing an unwitting example of the critique of essentialism, because everything can be treated as reversible under the auspices of the scientific imaginary. Just as one might object to the notion of reason, because the future might show its revisability as new developments occur, so did Walt Disney bristle at the idea of his death and its finality in the face of the great potential of future scientific research. Here, the idea of the world as an open book awaiting undreamt-of future discoveries plays the same card as other notions of immortality at which the same characters sneer. Plainly, both the hard-hearted and warm-hearted seem to want to live forever, but it is a curious objective that makes us wonder what such a situation would be like (for example, would we live as we are or be rejuvenated by an elixir?), that is, if we did live forever would it be as changing or unchanging?

Again, from the perspective of cryonics, life and death are the same insofar as they are simply examples of information, which is an old-fashioned way of treating life as textual, an object of desire, that is oriented to, even in death, which can be "read" in different ways. Interpretation (and hence research) is an ongoing infinite process of disclosing and codifying the world as if a text in ways that display present certainties. If the difference between life and death is "objective," then the passage between them is reversible in an ongoing way depending upon the contingencies of future research. Here, science accepts the Grey Zone by reducing it to the "object" of scientific exploration that changes over time. The ambiguity of what is known at any present is made to include death too in a way that makes ignorance relative and dependent upon "paradigms" of historical succession. But then knowing is identified with necessary skepticism towards what is known in any present as if it is this skepticism (based on the capacity to imagine anything thinkable) that is itself knowledge. If to have knowledge of anything is to imagine it being overturned, and so, essentially unstable, even this equation of fantasy with knowledge must depend upon the stability of a common language.

Death by Implication

The imaginary relation to death that life always seems to face takes its bearings from the ideal of necessity and its infraction, recognizing that there is no necessary or empirical relationship between life and death. This is to say that there exists no method of predicting or inferring anything about our death (that is, not how we will die, say, in agony, in bed, etc. but *our being dead*) from the kind of life we live. That is why we often try to imagine the conditions under which we will be dead, which is to say, how or whether our being dead might be animated (suggesting, curiously, that we might be dead and alive at the same time). We who live typically imagine that in being dead we will, at best if lucky, be an image.

> The cadaver is its own image. It no longer entertains any relation with this world where it still appears, except that of an image, an obscure possibility, a shadow ever-present behind the living form which now, far from separating itself from this form, transforms it entirely into shadow.
>
> (Blanchot [1955] 1982, 258, quoted in Schwenger 2000, 400)

Peter Schwenger develops Blanchot's connection between cadaver and image using decomposition as itself an image of the reputedly normal form of perception in life, a metaphor for the constant passage between subject and object in life (413). Death encourages the collective to imagine any life as an image to be used and developed according to any interests that prevail and are enforced. We who live imagine being dead as if an image in the hands of others, decomposed according to whatever passages between subjectivity and objectivity those who live after us suffer. Of course, there are methods for trying to guarantee such a connection, advanced often by religions, ethics, and (as the Wizard would say) doers of good deeds, but regardless of whatever values to which our life conforms and our repute attains, such values and our repute remain revisable, every bit as decomposable as our bodies themselves, as if our image is as vulnerable as our body to such a passage (or as Hegel says, the barbarians can come and destroy our temples, libraries, and archives, including revising the *persona* of the dead). In other words, it seems as if the difference between being alive and being dead makes reference to a border between what is under our control and not, as if when we are dead we are solely in the hands of others. But this begins to reveal a startling lesson of death, for this is not a difference: in life we are as much in the hands of others as we are in death. Death testifies to a conceit of life in this sense, that from the point of view of life, we always imagine being master of our fate in ways that, in death, we find unimaginable. Or to say it otherwise—whether in life or death we remain an image.

Being in the hands of others raises the question of the difference in my being a "utility," as used or used up, that is, my use value (how is anyone treated as a good or as Good, as a perishable that is consumed and extinguished, or as digested and excreted in ways that are transformative?). Death raises the question for anyone to ask of the others, just what uses do you intend to make of me, and do you even know, and to whom am I speaking anyway?

In a related vein, Steven Justice's paper (2008) on the belief in miracles in the Middle Ages resists the temptation to explain away such "superstition" by making it intelligible as a result of culture, social structure and the like, by inquiring into the commitment to false belief. Instead of treating such belief as socially constructed or as functional, he suggests that to believe in what might appear false (say, immortality in our case, or typically, to that for which evidence is lacking) can be a commitment to faith as a way of identifying with or imitating one's higher part. In contrast to the Enlightenment model of belief as superstition that can be made intelligible as functional or socially constructed, we can treat the believer as one doing self-arousal by seeing herself in the Other and the Other in herself, with the miracle an occasion for empowerment, i.e. believing it because it is wrong sustains her resolve as an actor. It is in this sense that I see the subject as performing at life in ways that I will develop later on in this book.

From time immemorial, people have tried to formulate a connection between one's life in the practices of living as one does (its content, "values") and how one will be responded to after her death, coming to the conclusion that there is no necessity in this relationship, that our life can make no guarantees, cannot determine what will be made of us, and because of this, stimulates us to create a range of imaginary connections that are (perhaps) necessary *and* hermeneutically challenged. Death then shows us something important about desire and its limits: if desire operates in life as a motor force animating all of our passages, death perhaps makes this clear and discloses the structure of such as a life force whose irresolution and unfulfilled character must withdraw and give space to the "fraught equivocation" (Didi-Huberman [1990] 2005) of the compulsion to live, to endure the possibility of impossibility. That there is no contractual relationship binding life and death can produce resignation, fear and trembling, nihilism, or a sense of anything whatever. It is normal to desire a connection, and in wishing for a connection, *any* connection, between life and death, we invariably confirm our seduction by a powerful force of life. In Baudelaire's idiom, jouissance can be understood as absolute for the subject insofar as laughter expresses "the delight we take in the image" (States 1995, 10–11) in the face of its division as useful, referential, as a likeness on the one hand (and so, relative in this way), and its corporeality on the other hand as a thing-in-itself, a site of beauty, a fantastic disfiguration (and so, as absolute in this way).

If such a connection could be supplied by the ways in which we relate to the death of others, and if every death of another provides us with a cadaver that, at the same time, must be animated much like the image, then relating to the death of the other is much like the relation to our dream upon awakening, to Freud's phenomenon of dream forgetting or to the remains of a dream destined to be fragmentary (Didi-Huberman [1990] 2005, 158). This makes the destiny of life as an object, fated to be dreamlike as an image, the life fated to be disseminated as fragments "as vestiges of (our) subjective being," not likenesses correlative with the name but in the manner of resemblances, of fantastic simulacra, perhaps even larger than the life that seems to evoke them, relating to the life as if a corpus marked not simply in the abundance of interpretations about the life but through the force of the fragment and in the persistence of this very fragmentation as the questions of the remainder, of the remains, and of remaining, of the passage of a life from object to image and to object itself as the story of remaining and of temporality as such, as the passage both and at once composed (absolute) and decomposed (relative) for any who would care to think, who would care for thinking. Thus, the three stages in Derrida's thinking on death, reflected as I suggested, in considering the death of others, the possible impossibility of one's own death, and the afterlife or dissemination, seem to mark the inevitable trajectory of the discourse as it passes through grief, fear and trembling, and the contemplation of oblivion, causing any writing such as this to wonder why it matters or, to paraphrase Lenin, what is to be done (and said).

> Then, in this supreme jeopardy of the will, art that sorceress expert in healing, approaches him; only she can turn his fits of nausea into imaginations with which it is possible to live. These are on the one hand the spirit of the sublime, which subjugates terror by means of art; on the other hand the comic spirit, which releases us, through art, from the tedium of absurdity.
>
> (Nietzsche [1886] 1956, 52)

If those such as Adorno suggest that we learn about death through life as we age, this remains the typical position of critical theory that treats reflection as caused by a degree of self-interest, in this case our aging making us think about death as if the body and its growing incapacity forces upon us such a reflection. In contrast, the convention of the Greeks and even Heidegger, certainly Freud and Lacan, make death topical for the human subject, as a condition of being human and oriented to this as such. If in this sense Freud shows quite well how this disregard must be oriented to as a condition of life and of its vitality, he nevertheless says that we do learn about death through our very mundane and routine experiences with loss and separation, even as we defer and need to bracket out the sense of death as our fatality. In a way, Freud, Schwenger, Heidegger, and these others treat life as so intimately bound up with the aesthetic impulse that the neutralization of death must be as if second nature and two-sided, if part of a narcissistic need to endure and enhance one's moment, and visible as if instrumental through and through because of this (as if I wasn't dying I wouldn't think of death!), yet still ambiguous as a phenomenon, revealing in its way the collective imaginary as arrested around the notion of instrumental action itself and its formulaic hold.

Basically, the mantra of the nihilist that everything is an image translates as the materialist credo, everything is a body, and so, perishable, imposing in this way a brake upon the enthusiastic gullibility of any initiative that aspires towards a final objective, suggesting that everything (like the body in Schwenger's example) is not simply a beginning but the beginning of decomposition. Since the image as a relationship to an (hypothetical) original is invariably the façade of whatever transpires in developing the relationship, the inevitability of decomposition reiterates that each beginning simply expires and never reaches finality in a way that makes life a series of unending beginnings. This repeats Nietzsche's conception of the universality of becoming. Yet life might also be refreshed by this notion of unending beginnings as a way of opening us to the unending series of actions it might promise and towards which it could lure us as those subject to the jouissance of development per se in the absence of the payoff.

Making sense of the cadaver, of the body, seeing it as a life, requires something beyond that connection, beyond the relation of the name to the activities and practices as if an obituary or biography, because that relation must be fundamentally ambiguous, reproducing the message of the primal scene for both (i.e. for the one who "reads" the life, and for the one whose life it is and was and who is seen-as in retrospect trying to interpret oneself and make his or her self legible through actions, who now, in our relation to such an one, must remain indecipherable in the way of the enigma of the primal scene). The cadaver seems like a memorial, repossessing in an impossible way the life it now emblematizes. And just as the cadaver cannot possess its past (only signify it), but then it never did, so it is fated to disappear itself just as the life it signifies, leaving only the traces that note its presence as something past that has passed. That the body too must perish allows us to appreciate the life as more than this, if we can, burdening memory with this task of perpetuation. But then if memory qualifies as such a monument, it, too, cannot stand forever. For the living who reflect, death always seems to take shape as a question of remains and of who and what will remain to care for the remains, and what and how might they do this and to what shall they be responsible and why. Who will remain with the remains?

Comedy and life affirmation coexist as a sign of the force that makes the desire to live laugh at itself, seeing the fool and their foolishness in the mirror, such plucky little creatures taking pleasure in what is bound to pass away! Such laughing at oneself can in the best of circumstances take shape in the hallucinating that speaks about oneself as two, speaking to the other as if we are two and one and speaking to another as if this is so, showing one's division as if (in) a dream, story, or film (as creator, director, and actor, commenting too), showing self-description as other than confession but as displaying one's contradictions as if the action of a fool (and not self-deprecating either), simply treating oneself as if a character in a narrative that one created for oneself out of the materials of one's life (made a life, wrote about a life). Such a dying one, at the point of death, might treat repossessing life as the work of a character in the play of life (taking *theatrum mundi* seriously). In this way, one treats the Real (life) symbolically by making (his/her) life a story and then reversing by making the story real in living and speaking it.

Outwitting the Nihilist

The first message of the nihilist is that the groundlessness of being allows us to do whatever, whether hedonism or inaction, because we are encouraged to see that there is no need to be accountable to anyone or anything. Derrida's reading of the Czech philosopher Jan Patočka brings out Patočka's notion of how religion in some way engages the demonic, where the secret refers to the trauma released by the fact of death and its mystery. Thinking about death and its implications can be liberating in this way, exempting us from heavy moralistic and self-indulgent constraints of external responsibility, or what Richard Florida calls burdens of the past. Strangely, remembering death does not have to depress us but can actually stimulate our creativity. Patočka criticizes the use of religion to act out or engage the unknown in irresponsible ways, in contrast to the notion of self-monitoring that he thinks that religion in the best sense makes possible. Derrida ([1992] 1995, 20) says:

> There is first of all demonic mystery in itself, one might say. Then there is the structure of secrecy that keeps that mystery hidden, incorporated, concealed but alive, in the structure of free responsibility that claims to go beyond it and that in fact only succeeds by subordinating mystery and keeping it subjugated… . In short, waking from demonic *mystery*, surpassing the demonic, involves attaining the possibility of the *secretum*, of the keeping of a secret. For it also involves gaining access to the individualization of the relation to oneself.

Durkheim identifies the mystery first in *The Division of Labor in Society* ([1893] 1933) in ways that make transparent the impossible and necessary desire for life, the mystery of this problematic desire for life, disclosing in this way life itself to be the mystery, and its demonic character to reside in the havoc this can create if the secret is not kept, keeping hidden but alive this secret while claiming to move beyond it. Durkheim shows how anomie works in its way to conceal the secret, and yet, to preserve it in some sense, as the action of being responsible to any present and its demands (see my discussion of death in Blum 2011a, 250–251; 2011b; 2012; 2014). Yet the nihilist urges that we do not have to accept the solution of the bourgeoisie to be productive and preoccupied, for we can be creative in any way we choose if we give up unrealistic versions of the self, if we relinquish beliefs that unsettle us. In this way, materialism treats the belief in a self as diseased insofar as it depends upon an impossible empirical conception of a tangible referent, and so, dismisses the phenomenon of hallucination by identifying it as phobic rather than as necessary and playful equipment for living.

Materialist Redemption

What Baudrillard calls Molecular Idealism emphasizes austerity as the paragon of productivity. Molecular Idealism imagines a new self and its manner and means of being productive in new ways. It is in the service of the productivity of this new self that the parsimonious relationship to meaning is directed and governed. In this sense, medical science as a regime seems to approximate what Lacan calls the discourse of the university with its emphases on productivity, objectivity, administrative rationality, performance evaluation, quantification and the like, and the attempt to humanize this beast in each and every area, for example as renewing subjectivity in medicine itself, as the discourse of hysteria in the cybernetic vision of a selfless self for everyone. It would seem from this perspective that the primary matter to engage or the real object to heed in the dementia caregiver's witnessing is the aporia of the dementia sufferer in relation to the fundamental ambiguity of life (its negativity in Hegel's sense) as a first startling encounter with the unknown as a futureless future to inhabit in the present. This is to say that the recognition of the unknowability of death is the commonplace way of coming to a recognition of the limits of life and its fundamental ambiguity (a recognition that can and could be conceded in any and every social relationship throughout a life) but that only death can make perfectly clear to many.

The materialist vision of life allows us to introduce the Lacanian use of the figure of the Moebius strip insofar as death is tangible and external and yet necessarily "internal" to life as a relationship to engage. This notion of the concrete universal translates the sociological recognition of any idea or abstraction as a course of action insofar as it (as a notion) has to be engaged as a representation "within" life despite its apparent externality. This invites us to consider a paraphrase of Lenin's question from another context—what are we to do? This is the question of care with respect to how we can imagine our comportment not simply towards the one cared for or the caregiver but to anyone and everyone (including oneself). In other words, besides succumbing to phobic obsession in relation to material conditions, what opportunities does life offer for creatively engaging death and material conditions? I started in these pages by reviewing various ways of putting (the thought of) death to rest, imaginable as religious, demonic, perhaps normal or neurotic as the solution of the bourgeoisie. Must we forget death or integrate it in some way in life? As I noted, Lacan speaks of adaptations to the Real such as repression, disavowal, and foreclosure in ways meant to distinguish neurosis from psychosis. If the "solution" of the bourgeoisie is neurotic, and the foreclosure in not being able to put death into words seems psychotic at first, the suffering of dementia might offer us another view. For example, in reviewing a book by Darian Leader on madness, Adam Phillips (2012, 18) remarks in another context: "people are doing something by being mad, and it can be something good. They can be involved in what Leader calls the 'proper work' of building 'a system of ideas as a response to their experience of collapse.'"

Innovative Relations to the Self

If materialism affirms the terror or abyss of the inevitable and inescapable condition, it says that there is no escape from anxiety over death unless the castrated self, exercised by antiquated and false visions that produce melancholic senses of loss and hopeless expectation, is renovated. On the one hand, false self must be weakened and its humanistic and idealistic yearnings purged, and on the other hand, such non-existent self, e.g. neurons, must be strengthened enough (neuronically? perhaps through medication?) to desire change and rehabilitation. Thus, the false consciousness of idealism and humanistic essentialism that is viewed as having produced the delusions of an eternal life must be discarded, while yet such change requires a force strong enough to engage such an elevated ideal as offered by the materialist interlocutor. A suspension of disbelief here will at least gain peace of mind. So the heirs of the medical discourse and, more fundamentally, of Lucretius, recognize that they have created a situation that needs relief and that paradoxically requires humanization, renewal.

An important feature of materialism is its parsimony towards ideas that it treats as gratuitous or as holding us back from commitment to life and productivity, leading it to engage regularly in intellectual housecleaning, discarding useless and obsolete fixations. The malleability of materialism must work this way constantly even in the face of mortality.

The opera *Death and the Powers* depicted a rich and powerful man giving himself to computerization for everlasting peace, and the film *The Diving Bell and the Butterfly* is typically cited as exemplary of the way materialism can redeem its morbidity, by offering the gift of a virtual life after conventional death, but only on condition that the perpetuity and autonomy of the brain is accepted as a replacement for the vestigial and antiquated notion of self and its "experience" of subjectivity. Here, the nihilist offer as the price of discarding the self in order to relieve the anxiety of death an offer that is hard to refuse, begins to frame the discourse of death more dramatically. The offer draws on a critique that holds that the brain's biology—its neurophysiology—is simply a computational phenomenon "that can exist in any kind of material … does not need … the mortal body"

(Palaprat and Hartouni 2011, 390). This idea that what is essential to the self is immaterial disputes the very idea of the self as gratuitous, and moreover descends from an honorable line of critique marked, for example, by Hume at its best.

> *Death and the Powers* invites us to imagine a future when an essential condition of human life—death—has been overcome, because an abiding production of western philosophy—the division of mind and body—has been resolved by technical ingenuity.
>
> (Palaprat and Hartouni 2011, 388)

Conclusion

What need be accepted is that the self as fiction or delusion actually worked to impede the tranquility required to face the Grey Zone on the grounds that the unsettling experience of life in its vitality and incoherent ambiguity is a pathological condition that needs remediation: "There is no stable biological 'I' in the brain … what you call a 'self' is not a source of mental experience; it is rather, an effect of mental processes: the sense of self in the act of knowing is … 'created' by the brain's representational capacities" (Damasio 1999). Thus, Dupuy ([1994] 2009), among others in this updated Skinnerian mantra, affirms the cybernetic regime as identifying thinking as computation "immanent to neurons that could be simulated without resorting to mental constructs."

Note that if the fiction of the self was always accepted as a necessary bit of equipment for living that has to be engaged with humor and flexibility, it was never treated as an empirical demonstration but as part of the necessary play form of humanity. However, at present, the interlocutor, say, the nihilist, says that our lifelong acceptance of this equipment is making us sick and that to live in tranquility requires that we pay the piper and agree to accept the nihilist offer for peace of mind.

References

Adorno, Theodor W. (1998) 2000. *Metaphysics: Concept and Problems*. Translated by Edmund Jephcott. Stanford: Stanford University Press.

Améry, Jean. (1968) 1994. *On Aging: Revolt and Resignation*. Translated by John Barlow. Bloomington: Indiana University Press.

Arendt, Hannah. 1958. *The Human Condition*. Chicago: University of Chicago Press.

Benjamin, Walter (1925) 1998. *The Origin of German Tragic Drama*. Translated by John Osborne. London: Verso.

Blanchot, Maurice. (1955) 1982. *The Space of Literature*. Translated by Ann Smock. Lincoln, NE: University of Nebraska Press.

Blum, Alan. 2003. *The Imaginative Structure of the City*. Montreal: McGill-Queen's University Press.

——. 2011a. *The Grey Zone of Health and Illness*. Bristol: Intellect Press.

——. 2011b. "Life, Death and the In-Between: The Duck/Rabbit and the Face of the Clown." In *Spectacular Death: Interdisciplinary Perspectives on Mortality and (Un) representability*, edited by Tristanne Connolly, 21–41. Bristol: Intellect Press.

Bonner, Kieran. 1998. *Power and Parenting: A Hermeneutic of the Human Condition.* New York: St. Martin's Press.

Damasio, Aldo. 1999. *The Feeling of What Happens*. New York: Harcourt, Brace and Co.

Derrida, Jacques. (1992) 1995. *The Gift of Death.* Translated by David Wills. Chicago: University of Chicago Press.

Didi-Huberman, Georges. (1990) 2005. *Confronting Images: Questioning the Ends of a Certain History of Art.* Translated by John Goodman. University Park, PA: Pennsylvania State University Press.

Dupuy, Jean-Pierre. (1994) 2009. *The Mechanization of the Mind: On the Origins of Cognitive Science*. Translated by M.B. DeBevoise. Princeton: Princeton University Press.

Durkheim, Émile. (1893) 1933. *The Division of Labor in Society*. Translated by George Simpson. New York: The Free Press.

Freud, Sigmund. (1917) 1957. "Mourning and Melancholia." In *Volume 11, On Metapsychology: The Theory of Psychoanalysis*, translated by James Strachey, 245–268. London: Penguin.

Girard, René. (1972) 1977. *Violence and the Sacred.* Translated by Patrick Gregory. Baltimore: The Johns Hopkins University Press.

Heidegger, Martin. (1935) 1959. *An Introduction to Metaphysics*. Translated by Ralph Manheim. Garden City, NY: Doubleday/Anchor.

Justice, Steven. 2008. "Did the Middle Ages Believe in Their Miracles?" *Representations* 103 (1): 1–29.

Lacan, Jacques. (1959–1960) 1992. *The Seminar of Jacques Lacan, Book VII: The Ethics of Psychoanalysis 1959–1960.* Edited by Jacques-Alain Miller. Translated by Dennis Porter. New York: Norton.

Laplanche, Jean. (1970) 1976. *Life and Death in Psychoanalysis*. Translated by Jeffrey Mehlman. Baltimore: Johns Hopkins University Press.

Nietzsche, Friedrich. (1886) 1956. *The Birth of Tragedy and the Genealogy of Morals.* Translated by Francis Golffing. Garden City, NY: Doubleday.

Palaprat, Étienne and Valerie Hartouni. 2011. "The Neural Subject in Popular Culture and End of Life." *Configurations* 19 (3): 385–406.

Phillips, Adam. 2012. "Shaky Ground." *London Review of Books* 34 (4): 17–18.

Pogue Harrison, Robert. 2003. *The Dominion of the Dead.* Chicago: University of Chicago Press.

Proust, Marcel. (1927) 2003. *In Search of Lost Time, or Remembrance of Things Past: Volume VI, Time Regained.* Translated by Andreas Mayor and Terence Kilmartin. Revised translation by D.J. Enright. New York: Modern Library.

Schwenger, Peter. 2000. "Corpsing the Image." *Critical Inquiry* 26 (3): 395–413.

States, Bert O. 1995. *Great Reckonings in Little Rooms: A Phenomenology of Theatre.* Berkeley: University of California Press.

Weber, Max. (1905) 1930. *The Protestant Ethic and the Spirit of Capitalism.* Translated by Talcott Parsons. London: George Allen & Unwin.

4 Fear and Likely Stories

Introduction

Plato's *Phaedo* remains the classical western text on death with Socrates arguing throughout that death is not to be feared because it is a blessed state insofar as we are freed from the body and its imperfections that create distortion and anxiety. Note that Socrates does not "prove" anything here as he is simply arguing about something of which he has no knowledge, basing his polemic upon an imaginary wish that a syllogism connects to the Real. The deep structure of his wish is imaginary not in the sense that he hopes to live forever but in his hope that a winning argument can convert ignorance into "truth." Not only is this a good example of the limits of an abstract relation to the world, it is also a gloss upon the collective representation of the body, ignoring the Grey Zone of corporeality (that the body can give us both pleasure and in many cases can even cause us to find pleasure in what gives us pain, e.g. self-destructive action, and pain in what gives us pleasure, e.g. guilt). This exposes the difference between a bad argument and faulty conceptualization, for it is not that he contradicts himself, but it is that he has no strong notion of a human subject and its relation to pleasure. Further, this seems to apply to his argument as well since he appears driven towards this belief in the force of argument. It is not that Socrates is illogical but that he seems delusional. Is the drive of philosophy to treat syllogism as eo ipso Real, not similar in its relentless single-mindedness to the thrust of the body and the imperativeness of the corporeal sense of drive? Could Plato be showing us the thin line between philosophy and psychosis that the fear of death can arouse in the human subject? Are humans not driven to fantasize their eternality, driven to wish for it as an addict might be driven? Even those many who have criticized Socrates here for his argument have typically accepted that epistemology is a reasonable way to engage death, saying (as Simmias and Cebes) that his argument is not compelling, instead of noting the absurdity of trying to "explain" death through epistemology. Yet, most do not recognize the limits of such an approach itself, that a reflective conversational approach to death does not mean that the speech must be ruled by this kind of idealization of the method of argument. To overcome an argument about death that appeals to empirical and logical evidence, we have to conceive of other alternatives, but perhaps Plato is disclosing such a path in his representation of the character of Socrates as a fool, as the one exemplifying Socratic ignorance, saying that in knowing that he is ignorant he is now committed in the present to affirm what he cannot know. Is Plato's fool possibly one who has the desire to fool around with empiricism and with empiricists by provoking them to reflect upon what they exclude in their beliefs and action?

Limits of Epistemology

In Lacanian, we could say that Socrates tries to fill the hole in Being (the space of the Grey Zone) with an argument in the expectation that the argument overcomes the "lack" (marked by uncertainty and a deficit in knowledge). Note that the argument itself is not satisfying and cannot be because its abstract notation on the relation of language to jouissance only discloses the unfulfilled status of desire. Fundamental ambiguity is best engaged by overcoming the temptation to view it as a lack by grasping its parameter as a condition of shared being and thus as a hole in Being. Note again in this case how Plato implies that it is conceptualization rather than such evidence that makes an account good or bad, that is, disclosing how the limits of the Socratic account can be seen in the way it engages the relation of mind to body that is implied in the notion of pleasure with Socrates appealing to an either/or model of the division that the discourse progressively unmasks. Plato suggests that to arm ourselves against fear we need a story that can supply the healing touch in ways that appeals to empirical evidence and syllogistic justification cannot. In centering attention upon the best story in a way that links it to healing, Plato relates narrative to health through the rhetorical gesture of a story that serves as equipment for living, the story that can best fortify us in a present to deal with the anxiety and resignation that death reveals as our fate. That is, we do not fail because we lack better knowledge about an afterlife or because we need to wait for science to provide some evidence. Rather, our "failure" consists in not engaging this ineluctable ambiguity as what Durkheim might call a normal social fact, as an essential aspect of the human condition that invites an antidote that heals rather than tries to find a cure. The criterion of truth is redefined from its concerns with correspondence or coherence to health, that is, to a concern for the conditions of speech that makes us better, healthier under such conditions.

Since the phenomenon being discussed is the fear of death rather than the behavior likely to occur in an afterlife, the account has to motivate all humans to find it compelling enough to continue at life in the present and to avoid distraction and demoralization.[1] As in a society ruled by theology where a syllogism might be compelling, or a scientific society disposed towards empirical evidence, Plato must rehabilitate the reputation of death for Greeks living a life in any present, giving them cause to see death as an image (a beginning) and not an original (an end) but to see it as a relationship to act upon in the present. Plato sees that life has to believe in death as not final, in order to give present meaning, and he does this through the notion of in medias res that demonstrates our influence by the dead. In other words, if we begin in the midst of an inheritance, we can be said to be influenced by the dead in ways that might give us incentive to regard our present actions as having this potential for influence upon the future. It is in this way that life comes from death as Cebes understands, and how the dead can be said to come back to life (in images, etc.), which Cebes doubts. It is as if the influences of death upon life can be accepted as part of the story of history but that this is not sufficient to silence the fear about the future and the worry about where the soul goes after the expiration of the body.

This fear according to Plato is based on the assumption that the relation of mind to body shows that they are both together and apart, divided and in relation. Materialism assumes an either/or relation where body rules mind in ways that can only confirm that the destruction of the body entails the destruction of the mind. If truly together, then they both die, but if they are apart how can their togetherness be demonstrated or preserved? Apartness seems to deny the influence of either upon the other unless we prioritize one at the cost of the other. Plato's solution is to see the relation as one of same to other where together is not the same as identical and apart is not the same as opposite, but similar and different in ways reminding us of the *aufheben*. Plato suggests that we need live life in ways that resist identity (seeing the body and soul as the same), as that can lead to hedonism and resignation, and that resist seeing the autonomy of each (as if the body and soul are opposites), as that can lead to asceticism. Plato shows that the opposition between fearing and not fearing death depends upon how we might think of fear in relation to mortality in any present and how best practices require some account that gives us strength to resist the extremes. The story then tries to formulate different ways of orienting to the fear of death by suggesting in its way that it is necessary and desirable in any present for one to conceive of having effects (on the future) *and* as being affected (by the past) or, in the words of Simmel, seeing that death bestows form-giving significance upon the present.

When the Winds Fail, Sailors Turn to Oars

The story reported in the *Phaedo* on Socrates' discussion of death with his friends is presented by Plato as if a history of that encounter that is reconstructed by an eyewitness. The eyewitness Phaedon was presented as such a witness. Note that the very topic of the *Phaedo* dramatizes the question of how we are to act in relation to temporal events for which there cannot be eyewitnesses, death in one case and most likely birth in other cases. Plato asks how we might formulate our relation to a future for which we lack an eyewitness in the present in ways that can give some satisfaction. Thus, we are at many removes from the referent, from death, from the discourse, from Plato, and Plato is removed from the event through the mediation of an eyewitness who represents the encounter, to we who read this as a story about the fear of death that is many removes from the events, their reports, or the climate and times of their occurrence, and in fact, to this text itself and its production and dissemination as an enigmatic moment in the great "chain of Being." Our lacking mastery of time deprives us of knowing death, just as our lacking knowledge of the discussion reported by Plato deprives us of knowing what transpired in the way that he lacks knowledge of the accuracy of Phaedon's recollection. We are mired in a landscape of mediation and intermediacy, exemplifying the perennially castrated human subject.

From his other works we can remind ourselves that Plato regards this as the lowest region of the divided line, imagination, in which we are ruled by images. Since the image presupposes a relationship to an "original" to which it responds in some way, a world ruled by images must be a world of unending relationships that are invariably beginnings. Plato uses the *Phaedo* to reveal death as an occasion to examine this kind of relationship to beginning, the primordial encounter of the human subject with the unknown as a beginning in which only informants and arguments seem to be resources for representation. Note how both the informant (here Phaedon) and the argument (of Socrates here), though fanciful, perhaps are the only ways of supplying material or usage for stories. Plato reveals that in the absence of eyewitnesses, abandoned only to informants and arguments, we need good stories that must artfully poach upon these very problematic accounts of the informants and of the arguments in order to develop. This best story, according to Plato, is able to appreciate both informants and arguments not as final but as a beginning with usage that enables working-through the collective speech. Can we say that Plato treats both informants and arguments as supplying "hearsay" not in the pejorative legal sense but as provocation (much like free association)? This requires us to see any argument as implicitly telling a story even as it conceals its idealization and any story as implicitly exposing its argument even as it pretends otherwise.

In an academic idiom, we say all arguments and stories are rhetorical. Thus any argument is grounded in the desire to relieve whatever gap it addresses in the way syllogism idealizes its proof, relations of entailment, and sense of trust in its other, just as any story conveys in its exposition an argument over the value of its method. In the way an argument is a means of motivation, so is a story an art for proceeding effectively under specific constraints. Just as the story is an argument and the argument a story, so is the informant (whether reliable or unreliable as they say in the cliché) one whose account can be interrogated not for its final solution but as a beginning, as an image that remains a provocation in the same way that the story and argument provoke rather than paralyze. Thus the content of the *Phaedo* as a beginning, an image, permits us to make explicit a circle of belief about the fear of death as usage that we might begin to take apart and work-through.

In contrast to Seth Benardete (2000, 292), I say that Plato's procedure is not ruled by the kind of syllogistic imaginary imputed here because this simply extends the authority of what Lacan calls the discourse of the university and its objectification of the text. It is not that we must see Plato seeking to test these hypotheses of the relation of body to soul in such a format that inventories and enumerates the propositions, if in contrast we recognize that he begins with the ambiguity of the relationship itself in a way that poses as a problem the question of its reconciliation, of the togetherness and apartness of body and soul, as a problem for working-through. Whereas Benardete suggests a Cartesian inventory in which Plato reads each proposition separately against the others in terms of a syllogistic model of the either/or, I suggest that the relationship that different participants strive to confirm or rebut is a discourse of adaptations to the fundamental ambiguity and irresolute character of this relationship that needs to be endured. The *Phaedo* asks us to imagine how we are to endure living with the irresolution of this question in a spirited way.

> Frivolous is not a bad word to sum him up ... if in the course of a lifetime he has done no significant harm, he has done no good either. He will leave no trace behind, not even an heir to carry his name. Sliding through the world: that is how in a bygone age, they used to designate lives like his: looking after his interests, quietly prospering, attracting no attention. If none is left who will pronounce judgment on such a life, if the Great Judge of All has given up judging and withdrawn to pare his nails, then he will pronounce it himself: A wasted chance.
>
> (Coetzee 2005, 19)

Pathos as an Affect

Living under the shadow of mortality in this sense suggests the need to engage waiting as something other than a test of endurance but, in some way, as incentive and opportunity that can seem both delusional and necessary. The necessity of delusion as such marks pathos as part of the human condition. If the affect of pathos must treat death as the deprivation of life that was possessed, melancholic adjustment to loss seems the only option for such a subject, searching for means and methods of relief. We want to begin to see such pathos as an affect that allows the subject to engage the life that is possessed as dispossessed, as inviting another kind of relationship, perhaps a way of addressing the jouissance of the life itself as a passage with other implications. We might begin to ask how the pathos of waiting and the boredom it inevitably raises can be acted upon as a situation requiring (indeed, inviting) something other than a phallic model of cure but a craft of healing. Admittedly, such an art must mix resources at hand in ways that are not simply detached but playfully engaged in the jouissance of this composing and fabricating, as if absorbed in and by its capacity to "make" a new kind of relationship under such conditions. Life in any present must be engaged as the making of jouissance, and so, as a kind of remaking of oneself. This requires overcoming the mix of sorrow and anger that leads to mechanical acting out. One way to understand those suffering under the sign of pathos is to hear them as asking for such an art, tempted by the extremes of resignation and longing mentioned by Simmel as primary affects, and the phallic solution of addiction that invariably seems intelligible. How can one who cares and who desires to exercise care for both oneself and any other hope to craft levity and lightheartedness in such a situation? Plainly, a gift of grace is required. The pervasiveness of pathos is recognized in David Foster Wallace's (2011, 143–144) fixation upon boredom.

> I'm talking about the fear that you and I have and that everybody has except nobody ever talks about it.... Our smallness, our insignificance and mortality,

> yours and mine, the thing that we all spend our time not thinking of directly, that we are tiny and at the mercy of large forces and that time is always passing and that everyday we've lost one more day that will never come back and our childhoods are over and our adolescence and the vigor of youth and soon our adulthood, that everything we see around us all the time is decaying and passing, it's all passing away, and so are we, so am I …
>
> And not only that, but everybody who knows me or even knows I exist will die, and then everybody who knows those people and might even conceivably have even heard of me or even knows I exist will die, and so on … and before maybe three or four generations it will be like I never existed, not only will I have passed away but it will be like I was never here …
>
> This is supposed to be news to us. News flash: We're going to die.
>
> Why do you think people buy insurance?

His example suggests that resistance to suicide requires boredom touched by melancholy to be converted into mourning. What is mourned is not the past or the future (loss) but the lack of imaginative vitality in any present (Deleuze's [1995] 2005, 18), in other words, the lack in and of commitment and the need for its renovation. Here we begin to identify the affect of pathos as an opportunity for reformulation and translation into some version of the jouissance and commitment to end-of-life that might invite replies other than futility.

This universality of pathos is masked by the illusion of the conquest of time, that we can have influences upon a future, revealing not the priority of biological disintegration in aging, for example, but the ways worldly attachments begin to recede in meaning as consequential with the passing of time, invariably weakening a subject who inevitably must start to lose a capacity for defense against the recognition of mortality and the pathos that must enter in the present scene of life.

The conception of pathos as what Durkheim would call a normal social fact allows us to see boredom both as malaise and as an occasion for healing. As in any disturbance such as this a further question asks if we can heal boredom (as addiction) through the method of symptom management or, in contrast, if we are driven to try to track its sources. If addiction is reputed to relieve boredom, the prior question asks after the grounds of boredom as a question that we might demand of ourselves as a matter of concentration and wonder despite its irreparability. It seems as if the notion of depression exists at this interpretive border. I am now posing the question—what form can palliative care take for reflective persons, that is, for those who are immune to banal stimulation? As Wallace points out, such care would have to be directed to the malady of boredom. The model of criteria for effective healing suggests that we explore the conditions for investing affect in a present as consequential and, at this point in our exposition, can lead us to query the proposition of whether art is capable of healing boredom or better, how an aesthetic relationship to the present might be good medicine for such a task. We can suggest further that the aesthetic relationship to the present serves in our model at present as the interlocutor to symptom management in the discourse on cure and healing.

> To speak of an aesthetic dimension of knowledge is to speak of a dimension of ignorance which divides the idea and the practice of knowledge themselves… . The object of aesthetic apprehension is characterized as that which is neither an object of knowledge nor an object of desire.
>
> (Rancière 2006, 1)

That is, to apprehend death aesthetically is not to see it in terms of its causal structure, material composition, nor as desirable or not, for these conditions that apply to the social representation of death do not evoke its intimate singularity, its "who" rather than what. To say that "aesthetic apprehension of a form is without concept" echoes Simmel's injunction to provide form to material conditions, to rethink the phenomenon not in terms of its efficiency or desirability, but as a representation accompanied by a certain ignorance (that is, knowledge of one's limits or in Lacan, of the hole in the symbolic order as a modernization of the maxim of Socratic ignorance). In this way, Rancière after Lacan and others finds oppressiveness not in death per se but in these ways of representing death (as knowledge, as undesirable) that neutralize an aesthetic relationship to speech. Thus, if a conventional view of death limits or "neutralizes" the element of desire in aesthetics, aesthetics then overcomes and elevates such views, "neutralizing" them in its way.

> It is thus that such experience is much more than appreciating works of art. It concerns the definition of a type of experience which neutralizes the circular relationship of knowledge as know-how and knowledge as the distribution of roles. Aesthetic experience eludes the sensible distribution of roles and competences, which structures the hierarchical order.
>
> (Rancière 2006, 4)

He says that the aesthetic experience "neutralizes" conventional speech just as I say that unreflective versions of death "neutralize" the aesthetic desire but we are saying the same: the aesthetic relation to speech "takes on wings" as Plato would say, readjusting, reallocating, and revitalizing the empty speech with which it begins and that holds it down with its restricted economy of signifiers. Thus, as the poetic impulse struggles with its own repressed core, it is through this "struggle" that the repressive structure of common speech is moderated, relaxed, revisited.

Art performs at life as if it matters insofar as even the representation of the malaise of characters in a novel or play or the ecstatic exhibition of action in any sort of theatrical is like the staging of a gaze of witnessing that invests the spectacle with the reassuring eye of a witness who knows and understands the most forlorn situation. Again, in Annie Baker's *The Flick*, the act of homage consists in the play's commitment to witness the struggle in desperation in its representation, making the voice of art and its capacity to see-as omnipresent in its power to see and witness such suffering in exhibiting it as a performance for those who very well might not see. For example when I saw Baker's play in New York, the audience treated it as stand-up comedy for most of the night until confronted with what they could not avoid, stopping their guffaws when the suffering reached its climax.

Self-Preservation/Primary Narcissism

Art and the relationship and motivated course of action it signifies, like any worldly preoccupation, cannot "solve" the problem of death for us but represses it in the tangled connections it revives and risks unravelling about us and for us as the experiential web in which we are enmeshed. We work through this web of desire by first managing the particular conditions that are registered in the stigma we inherit as if our birthmark, our insignia or identity. Second, in coming to recognize this mark as the image of the trauma of ambiguity and the loss of innocence that all suffer and ourselves in particular, we try to work it out through the weaving of connective tissue that emerges in our symptom. Then at best, we learn through critical moments and enigmatic collisions to read this symptom as the fiction of our story but of our making, in ways that tempt us to manage its disturbances or translate it as our part of a whole picture of relating to effects of common problems. We are eventually driven to renovate the symptom as if a strategy for enjoying its ambiguity, learning to incorporate it into our present as a tool felt as both oriented and automated in ways that equip us for living in the present. Death can cause us to ask of ourselves—if we agree that we want to live in the present—how should it be done?

In these ways, pathos correlative with the march of time cannot easily be rectified by techniques and in most cases cannot be easily detected by those without respect for its force as an influence upon the subject. Self-help advice, neurological information, or technically oriented palliative care cannot help a subject orient to those identified as vulnerable, for if the pathos of the subject is such a parameter, stimulated of course but not caused by vexation and bodily disabilities, healing must take other forms and be grounded in other sorts of relationships to the present of the subject. The next part of this book addresses this problem for the caregiver of the subject of age-related dementia, but uses this case as a matheme of the problem of care for any human being.

The relationship of materialism to mortality that we discussed earlier has long been recognized as imagining our inevitable limitation in the body. But we note also that its dedication to a notion of malleability can lead us to imagine even our bodies as endlessly revisable and open to change, suggesting here the bare possibility of conquering time and mortality. This assumption always risks identifying malleability with what has been called plasticity as a limited version of the notion. Indeed, this could be one view added to the corpus of understandings on how humans are reputed to differ from animals, not by virtue of suffering, which is shared, but by the capacity to convince oneself that immortality is possible. If it has been suggested that children and animals maintain their innocence in this respect, it might be proposed that humanity knowing this fact that it is mortal also hopes for a cure, revealing this loss of innocence as both betrayal and grounds of anger. Pathos signifies this mix that constitutes the environment of the wide-awake social actor, the experience of having been expelled from paradise.

The Value of Life

Such malleability is reflected in the corpus of opinions, beliefs, and stories intent on calculating the value of life. What we can engage in any present is a mosaic of such beliefs that we might revise, interrogate, and recreate as a tapestry of meanings. Here we begin to situate ourselves and our place in relation to the discourse on death and of course life, a discourse enveloping us as if a web of significance. We ask what can we learn from the spider caught in the web. Let us play with different voices in this collective speech. We imagine first the materialist voice and then the antidote that asks if art and the imagination can be expected to heal the anxiety of the spider.

Actuarial Death—Lawyer's Math in Sept. 11 Deaths Shows Varying Values for Life

By William Glaberson

The salesman was running late that morning. He called his wife to say he was probably going to miss his meeting at Windows on the World. But at the last minute, at 8:47, he called his office to say he had made it to the restaurant.

One minute later, American Airlines Flight 11 hit the building, the north tower of the World Trade Center. It was 100 minutes before the tower collapsed. He was 29.

The other day, a lawyer for the salesman's 27-year-old widow pushed back in his chair at a Park Avenue law firm and estimated how much the dead man's final suffering high over Manhattan might be worth one day in court. In another case a few years ago, he said, a jury awarded $365,000 to the survivors of a passenger who experienced five minutes of terror as a damaged plane careened to earth.

"You're talking about many minutes," the lawyer, James P. Kreindler, said matter-of-factly. "It should be a large award." Maybe $1 million, he said, for the salesman's final anguish.

Such calculations are being considered by hundreds of lawyers as they measure the potential value of cases of those who lost loved ones at the World Trade Center, the Pentagon and in the four hijacked planes.

The lawyers are asking uncomfortable questions. How much did the dead man make? Was the death fast or slow? Were the passengers terrorized by seeing flight attendants stabbed? How hot was the fire?

For centuries, civil lawsuits have tried to answer such questions in dispassionate economic terms. The main goal of a wrongful death suit is to replace financial support to the dependents of a person whose death was the result of an intentional act or negligence. In measuring the value of a lost life, lawyers often say that dollars are inadequate, but that they are all there is. In addition to damages for economic losses, intangible things, like the suffering before an inescapable death, are given a price tag. Lawyers say they are struggling to analyze how such intangibles should be computed in the Sept. 11 attacks.

[…]

In court, a lifetime of lost support is typically estimated through the testimony of economists. By analyzing age, salary, and other benefits, they project how much a person might be expected to earn over a lifetime.

From that sum is subtracted the amount the person might have spent on things like subway fare or country club dues.

An economist might persuade a jury, Mr. Kreindler argued, that a hard-driving person like the salesman might work well past 70. It was plausible, he said, to assert that the salesman would have had 40 years ahead of him and that he would have earned more than $500,000 in each of those years. In all, the lawyers concluded, the economic losses might be as much as $25 million.

[…]

A few days after the lawyers computed what the salesman's case fight bring, another lawyer, Alan L. Fuchsberg, was estimating the value of a case involving another man who died on Sept. 11.

He was 42 and earned $54,000 as a clerk in a financial firm in the World Trade Center.

Mr. Fuchsberg said the clerk's case might bring a substantial award for pain and suffering. The office he worked for was on the 90th floor of the second tower to be hit, where there were announcements encouraging people to return to their desks while the first tower burned.

The clerk, Mr. Fuchsberg said, would have had plenty of time to understand his circumstances. "Obviously," the lawyer said, "it got very smoky and hot and unbearable."

But Mr. Fuchsberg said he told the clerk's father to expect a comparatively small award for economic damages, especially if it was difficult to prove that the clerk, who was single, provided substantial support to his aging parents. Mr. Fuchsberg said some claims for single people with no dependents could be worth as little as $100,000. The clerk's father, who asked not to be named, said he was stunned to learn the role a person's income played in lawyers' math. "The value of a life is certainly not determined based on earnings," he said, his voice breaking. "We're talking about my son."

A Lawyer's Worksheet

How lawyers estimate the value of a wrongful death claim for a breadwinner:

Projected annual earnings × Expected number of years remaining of working life

+ The value of other expected income from the deceased person's labors.

– The amount that would have been consumed by the person who died, like expenditures for food, clothing, and personal hobbies.

+ The economic value of the deceased person's contribution to the household, like gardening work and driving children to school.

+ Compensation for nonfinancial losses suffered by the person who died, like the pain and suffering endured by the person because of the injury that caused death.

+ In some states, the value of the nonfinancial losses suffered by family members, like the loss of love and companionship for a spouse or the loss of parental care by a child.

Total:

Your Money or Your Life

If there is a randomness in the relation of life to death, then the life we live very well might have no relation to the way we are treated after dying, suggesting that we are as likely to lack effects as to have influence, that what we do and accomplish can be dissolved as if grains of sand. This view of a relation between life and death as external, as if death is a final act that deposits a life in the hands of others to do with as they wish, is the frightening prospect against which wishful thinking might seek to fortify itself. This makes *not* doing such wishful thinking the *sine qua non* of realism as if the unfriendly question ("Your Money or Your Life") posed by English robbers in the Middle Ages (Morris-Reich 2002, 131) was a reality test designed to confront idealists and humanists alike: that one must either renounce her abstract principle or die is meant to challenge the subject to "put up or shut up" by seeing whether she shall treat what she claims to believe as worth this risk, whether she has the courage of her convictions or has lived a life of phoney-baloney (see Blum 1996). Here, we might renounce wishful thinking and accept the gloomy prospect of the random relation of life to death. On the other hand, we might note that the "principle" is not the wishful thinking per se (as if the rule to be renounced is a deluded view of the afterlife), but the demand to "give up" a commitment to principle as such. That is, what the robber wants us to renounce is the commitment to the imaginary connection between the life we live and its influences and, consequentially, he wants us to give up the notion that life matters in the face of such randomness. The robber wants us to be good positivists and renounce life on the grounds of evidence that after death we are in the hands of others. This demand misrecognizes wishful thinking by treating it as an empirical prediction or as a need for reassurance "despite all facts:" in contrast, as the Greeks might say, wishful thinking desires any help and support it can get (from the Gods) to sustain a commitment to life, it prays or wishes for such inspiration to keep it going as the belief in life in the face of its recognition of fortuna, of the external relationship of life to death.

Actually, the choice in the robber's question between our money or our life is not really a choice if we understand the question to be about priorities. If money stands for what is most important to and for us, will we renounce this at the cost of dying? But if what is most important is integral and indispensable to a life, to give it up is to give up one's life. If the robber says that we can stay alive but without what is most important, we reply that that is not a life but death. On the other hand if we refuse to renounce what is most important and become dead, there is no guarantee that our renunciation will live in the future. So, we are facing two alternative deaths and not a choice between life and death.

In the canon, being willing to die has been treated both as a mark of heroism (die for principle) and as a kind of abstract selfishness, but always dependent upon what is most important. It is as if the willingness to die is taken as a test of the authenticity of our commitment. Here, sacrifice also enters as we recall Agamemnon, Abraham, and the line of martyrs, even leading up to Karl Schmidt's notion of friendship and death as a badge of commitment. Your money or your life seems to trade off the materialistic imaginary of skepticism reflected in the cliché "there is no atheist in the foxhole," or the reputed Mafia mantra "here is an offer that you cannot refuse!" So, regardless of the content, for believers and non-believers alike, the willingness to face being dead seems the best test of whether someone is on the up-and-up, always ready and able to expose the pretence of a life claimed to be centered by commitment.

The idea haunting this discourse, that we are prepared to relinquish what is important to us when faced with desperate circumstances, is what I think of as the "when push comes to shove" notion that we are ready to do whatever is required when threatened with death, and the element of truth here should not obscure the way such a vision functions in collective life to dishonor commitment and principle as if in the collective there must remain a constant animus towards the willingness to live with spirit and without illusion, to live with spirit precisely *because* of the absence of illusion, in the face of the material condition and irrevocable nature of our mortality (Blum 1996). Nietzsche alone caught this hatred towards those who commit to rebirth, to living life over and again with passion while knowing full well that they will die. Of course, Socrates demonstrated this in formulating the accusation against him at his trial and, instead of relinquishing his principle, employed it in defending himself.

Deconstructive Death and the Last Word: Derrida on Lacan

The example of Derrida's reconstruction of his relationship to Lacan elevates the discourse from the actuarial model of death and the empirical skepticism of ordinary views by its trying to speculate on the "meaning" of the relationship between associates as a way of determining the value of a life and the need for a robust aesthetically oriented story. Derrida creates an opportunity for such an engagement when he muses upon his historical relationship to Lacan in a way that both disavows and claims superiority while demonstrating a commonness in the face of the alleged and the elsewhere. That is, while Derrida ([2000] 2002) asserts the inevitability of alibi, of indirection, of making reference to making reference, of otherness, otherwhere, and elsewhere, to allegedness (xvii), at the same time he seems to exempt his own usage from such a disavowal, setting up the distinction between the proper and improper alibi (xvii: the difference between paralysis and aporia), comically ("strategically" his admirer would say) mixing his claim to superiority (to knowing the difference between aporia and paralysis) with the inevitability of inexorable indirection (just like everyone). While this is necessary and a comic condition in practice, Derrida shows deconstruction and its playful relation to language to inhabit the voice of ordinary (significative) humor from which comedy needs to develop.

In this respect, it is worth retelling Derrida's report on his encounter with Lacan, on the occasion of one of their few meetings at a dinner given by Lacan's in-laws, at which as part of the story, Lacan embellishes some incident in a narrative that includes naming Derrida "the father" in a way that seems both curious and worthy of thought to Derrida, who proceeds to speculate on why Lacan names him as such. In Lacan's narrative the father was identified as one who failed to recognize the way he "disregarded the Other by playing dead" as if playing dead is not only a failure to recognize Other but a failure to recognize that one is failing to recognize (i.e. not remembering that he is not remembering). But this is itself curious for it is this problem that inspires the book *Without Alibi* (the failure to remember we are not remembering) that appears forty or fifty years after this dinner without a mention of the puzzle and the debt, and further, seems to attribute in this double negation the failure to remember the failure to remember (that is, the unethical sense of alibi), to Derrida himself, by calling him "the father." Derrida ([1996] 1998, 51) of course wants to pursue the question of both what and who is the father here.

> Lacan's phrase speaks of a "father" and that's me, a father who "does not recognize … the way he disregarded the Other (big O) by playing dead… . I am still not sure I have fully understood the ventured interpretation … but I have always wondered whether by making me out to be the father in this story, by naming me "the father," he was not taking aim at the son; I have always wondered whether he didn't mean to say the son, if he didn't want to play the son, to make me or himself into the son, to make of me the son who disregards the Other by playing dead, as he put it, or make himself into the son. As always, Lacan left me the greatest freedom of interpretation, and as always I would have taken it even if he had not left it to me.
>
> (51)

What is immediately funny is that Derrida might be using the idiom of homage and of love for Lacan as a pretext for settling scores and for having the final word on who is the best man. Derrida leaves unspoken an account of the homage as an event and how it is made eventful in the cut, which it both conceals and intimates through the artifice of praise and gratitude that feigns behind indivisible speech what could be otherwise. What is striking in the homage to a dead person is that the living get the last word. It might be seen here how a concern for immortality as shared by Derrida and his collaborator Kamuf might (in their own terms) produce the usage of justice as a way of assuming (allegedly) its own value to depend on what lies elsewhere "for all the living and all the dead, past and yet to come" (Kamuf 2002, 21) as a speech intrinsically problematic, possibly unjust and self-serving, and certainly worthy of interrogation. Here we might have the last word.

If I also take advantage of such a freedom of interpretation, let me propose first that Derrida uses the homage to work out his concerns for his relation to Lacan, using sibling rivalry to gloss a discourse about dissemination, influence, and posthumous perpetuity. First suggesting that Lacan's naming him, Derrida, the father who disregards Other (which could be disparaging and insulting) seems to show for Derrida Lacan's sense of Derrida as the son who disregards the influence of the father as if Lacan is admonishing Derrida for disregarding his own influence, the fatherly influence of Lacan (as if the old goat Lacan is treating Derrida defensively and as an adolescent). Thus, Derrida interprets Lacan as naming him, Derrida, the father, as a device that could disguise his fear of Derrida as a rebellious son who eschews the influence of his father. But note that Lacan *does* call Derrida the father and can mean it with every right (and here Derrida is taking the same liberties in misreading Lacan that he regularly admonishes us for doing in our interpretations). This permits Derrida to treat Lacan as the angry father whose influences are not honored, and to treat himself as the free spirit (exemplified in the end of this excerpt in Derrida's self-description of himself as unbound as such, and more darkly in Lacan's premonition that Derrida, having the last word, might be less free than self-indulgent). That is, what if Lacan names Derrida the father who disregards Other and implies himself as the son for good reason, suggesting perhaps not only that deconstruction will "do as it pleases" by exercising its freedom to appropriate the oeuvre as it sees fit, but more pertinently that Derrida as the father personifies that voice of interdiction that qualifies any resolution and, in its way, threatens to steal the jouissance of desire, of the aesthetic imperative, by reminding *it of its eternal deconstructibility* as if it is this reminder that is fearless as such ("without alibi") rather than, say, the desire to proceed in the face of such deconstructive reservations, the desire to take such a risk (without alibi). In this way, Lacan reminds Derrida that if his philosophy "plays dead" by using the alibi of being "without alibi" it can only be in disregard of Other, which requires of any action that it accepts its allegedness without alibi. In other words, Lacan might be accusing the father of lying to himself (in ways that Derrida and Peggy Kamuf find "philosophically incoherent" in Arendt). Thus, we could use the "freedom of interpretation" disseminated by an oeuvre not simply to show the fundamental ambiguity of this exchange ("to do as we please") but to hint at other stakes involved in talk as such, stakes involving the question of control over means of interpretation.

This is why I am proposing without alibi that Lacan is impersonating Plato (who is reputed to have asked about Aristotle's absence from a meeting "where is nous?" i.e. where is the one we might call "mind," the one who sets himself up as the paragon of pure thought), by calling Derrida "the father," i.e. the one we might call "interdiction," the one who sets himself up as the last intellectually honest man, Mr. Reminder, the one whose playing at being dead not only disregards Other but steals the jouissance of human desire. In other words, Lacan is calling Derrida an obsessive whose "disregard" of Other is animated by a fear for its volatile potential. Here perhaps Lacan surmises of the future imagined by Derrida, the Derridean imaginary, as follows: if what we share is the opportunity to take and to give "freedom of interpretation," what differentiates us can only be the specific use we make of such freedom (what we say and do), the unending circulation and contact of pleasure and interpretation, of the future "doing as it pleases" with whatever comes its way as interpretable, in a view of eternity as hermeneutically fecund in ways only threatened by the tyrannical gesture that would not grant such freedom, or by the unimaginable absence of productivity, the lack of materials upon which we can exercise our freedom. The only obstacles to this landscape of posterity is the wasteland as such. In contrast, Lacan introduces the notion of a healing art through his conception of the fantasy released by the drive of libido as equipment for living.

> That which lies beyond is not simply the relationship to the second death or, in other words, to man to the extent that language demands of him that he realizes the following, namely, that he is not. There is also the libido, that is to say, that which at fleeting moments carries us beyond the encounter that makes us forget it. And Freud was the first to articulate boldly and powerfully the idea that the only moment of jouissance that man knows occurs at the site where fantasms are produced, fantasms that represent for us the same barrier as far as access to jouissance is concerned, the barrier where everything is forgotten.
>
> (Lacan [1959–1960] 1992, 298)

Lacan's naming Derrida the father might just be a way of calling into question the interdiction upon aesthetics in the name of ethics, and here Derrida taken to personify the censorious voice of a philosophy that would always remind us that enthusiasm needs to be regulated. The father who plays dead and will do as he pleases suggests that to play dead is to act as if immune to stimulation (compelled by rigor) and a refusal to be charmed or manipulated, as if driven by righteousness or whatever, to abide by his decision not to be charmed or influenced. This could be proposed playfully if we imagine Lacan thinking that he said everything before Derrida, insulated in the formula of das Ding, leaving Derrida to deconstruct such formulae by pointing out lacunae in speeches (for example, why only three registers of imaginary, symbolic, real?), and disclosing deconstruction as such a capacity to note limitation in any signifier as a kind of phobic obsession. In this sense, Lacan could be seen not at all as Derrida suggests, but as one who reveals the father as parasitic in the way admonishment depends upon its victims. Perhaps Lacan is admonishing Derrida then, as the father who plays dead could very well be pointing out that admonishing (as fathers do) is never enough, that the interdiction as it stands is not creative and risks playing dead rather than making something bound to suffer ambiguity and deconstructability.

Imagination and the Value of Life: Ignominy, Memory, and the Archive as a Fantasy

The fantasy that "carries us beyond the encounter … that makes us forget it," what Lacan calls after Freud, libido, is a suggestive way of formulating our engagement in the present. Libido is akin to what Simmel conceived as the two-sided nature of desire as part of life and as reaching beyond for "more than life." Libido then resonates not with desire and an expectation of phallic fulfillment but with the insistence of what Lacan calls drive and its almost corporeal imperativeness as if a demand for more than life. Indeed, this is how Durkheim formulated the Grey Zone of life as the environment of one subject to an awareness of mortality that I used at the beginning of this work. Libido identifies the necessity of such a dream.

We might now appreciate the missing element in the Socratic story that we examined earlier in this chapter, for his anxious concern for existence in time seemed to leave out the libidinal character of the story, its hallucinatory but necessary character. In other words, Plato's Socrates was made to revel in his ignorance perhaps as a device to exhibit the necessity of such poetry as equipment for living, in this sense, made to play the fool in life. Socrates, like Freud much later, knew the value of such stories as a confirmation of human malleability without respect to their truth or falsity. Note H.D.'s reflection on Freud, "the Professor."

> "Eros and Death, those two were the chief subjects-in fact, the only subjects-of the Professor's eternal preoccupation. They are still gripped, struggling in the deadlock. Hercules struggled with Death and is still struggling. But the Professor himself proclaimed the Herculean power of Eros and we know that it was written from the beginning that Love is stronger than Death. It was the very love of humanity that caused the Professor to stand guardian at the gate. Belief in the soul's survival, in a life after Death, wrote the Professor, was the last and greatest fantasy, the gigantic wish-fulfillment that had built up, through the ages, the elaborate and detailed picture of an after-life. He may even have believed this. If so, it was proof again of his Centurion courage. He would stand guardian, he would turn the whole stream of consciousness back into useful, into irrigation channels, so that none of this power be wasted."
>
> (H.D. 1956, 103)

Despite his scepticism towards the content and detail of such stories, Freud recognized the necessity of this libidinal force in life. Yet if the stories never made explicit beliefs about the value of life, according to Freud they seemed to affirm that value as connected to the malleability of human expressiveness.

Van Haute uses the exchange "How much is a life worth … lots and lots of money" (Van Haute 2002, 167) as an example of the void as an object as in Wittgenstein's notation on the irresolute search for the "essence" of a matter that is analogous to the notion of the "signifier of a lack inherent in its very function as the treasure of the signifier," the subject always in-between (Van Haute 2002, 171). The dream of the value of our life in the present relates to Lacan's conception of libido as fantasy that helps us forget what we mean (in using the cliché inflexibly as a metonym) and to remember that we forget when we study it (in using the cliché metaphorically).

There, he assumes that living is a kind of choice and oriented in its way, but basically (and as I note in that text) the continuation of life seems to be more like a drive, almost compulsive and not as if a freely chosen option, leading us to begin to understand the automated character of social conduct as mixing body and mind in the notion of jouissance or of the sensual engagement with the moment, and in this way as a reflection of the force that both Freud and Lacan wanted to develop. So the spider drives to go on and to make and enjoy a story that can sustain such a path with a degree of sexual finality that is not phallic but consummatory in its play, needing a kind of ribald engagement with images, conduct, and language. If Durkheim suggests that life itself and its continuation is a habit, we need to grasp the tactility of such habituation, partly through the metaphor of "going on," of motive in the strongest sense or affect.

I have suggested elsewhere that jouissance in the present lives in part through a conception of one's singularity as inscribed in the archive of moments said to constitute one's memory. Derrida among others has shown the force of the spectral and the ghosts of the past in the present in his exploration of Freud, and I am proposing now that the engagement with and in the present as an opportunity for jouissance "carrying us beyond the encounter," and in its way making us capable of forgetting it, is worked-out in our use of this archive in the present. If it is this unshareable archive of impressions that marks us to ourselves as singular, our memory must be an opportune curriculum for us in the present. In this way the lived experience of any dying body must be seen to include such a narrative propensity, an inarticulate struggle to represent and reflect upon the history of erotic turning points or "adventures" that mark the movement of its life and indeed of any life. Care requires an open capacity to witness this madness.

The importance of memory in the lived experience of the dying body is its character as an archive of traces commemorating or marking the moments of a life. Thus, collecting mementos, whether possessions, things, memorabilia and the like has been treated as obsessive hoarding or as penury, but can also be seen as the drive to keep alive one's sense of singularity as if its extension into the unknown future will be conveyed by the things amassed. In this way memory depends not only upon the past and the discrimination exercised to make a collection out of the unruly remains, but on the future as well and the conversation and uses imagined in the capacity of unknown others to endow what is left with value. The archive, combining the intimacy of past remains with the anonymity of future uses is embodied in the anxiety of memory and its need to dwell in any present on what it has and/or possesses and how this can be maintained and protected from loss or distortion.

Conclusion

When Freud says that forgetting death requires repressing repetition and inevitability, he means that we repress the past as the determinant of the present, and so, circularity, and we repress the future and our inexorable death, and so, its relevance to our present, rejecting both the possibility of learning from the past and of influencing the future. This means that what we "really" repress is the fact that we live only in the present, and we accept the delusion that our time is eternal, with the sense of repetitiousness and inevitability being reminders of this circularity. As the novelist William Faulkner says in *The Sound and the Fury*, to fail to remember in this sense and to open ourselves to the delusion of our time as absolute is akin to the fools who try to conquer time (Blum, 2014). Yet the novelist might be shortsighted here for the "fools" can also be seen as those who commit to perform at life as art and its "as-if" as consequential, the "as-if" reflecting an aesthetic drive to live life as if it matters, an artful gesture that exposes at the foundation of life the need to perform at living in accordance with Nietzsche's conception of life as aesthetic at its core. So in Baudelaire's sense of absolute comedy, it could actually be Faulkner's fools who feign acting as if they are aspiring to conquer time, and so, seem to be as if unaware of their limits and who in doing so only appear to pursue the worst knowing the best, but actually pursue the best while knowing the worst (performing at life knowing mortality, accepting the deceit and knowing that they do). This is the "courage" many insist that life requires, the courage to be playful towards the present by performing at it as if it matters while knowing full well that its fate to pass away makes any such stance both necessary and hallucinatory. The hallucination in this sense is a dream. This drive towards the dream is also the spine of Kenneth Burke's conception of equipment for living. Thus, the whiff of egoism is always raised by suicide in giving pause to our habitual tendency to see surviving life at any cost the *sine qua non* of instrumental action (the figure of the survivalist), because suicide can and often does lead us to see taking one's own life, curiously, as an egoistic gesture, since in wanting to quit the rat race and leave life in order to have peace of mind it refuses to make the sacrifice demanded of life. This is a question and not a conclusion.

Note

1 Actually, there are those reputed now to speculate on the afterlife, even "hard" scientists, probably fortified by their piety towards science, who desperately want to imagine living forever. See Brian Bethune (2013), "The Heaven Boom."

References

Baker, Annie. 2014. *The Flick*. New York: Theatre Communication Group.
Benardete, Seth. 2000. "On Plato's 'Phaedo.'" In *The Argument of the Action: Essays on Greek Poetry and Philosophy*, 277–296. Chicago: University of Chicago Press.
Bethune, Brian. 2013. "The Heaven Boom." *Maclean's* May 13, 44–48.
Blum, Alan. 1996. "Fear and Panic: On the Phenomenology of Desperation." *The Sociological Quarterly* 37 (4): 673–698.
——. 2014. "Guide for the Perplexed: Science and Literature as Equipment for Living (In Preparation)." *Philosophy and Rhetoric* 48 (1): 54–72.
Coetzee, J.M. 2005. *Slow Man*. New York: Viking.
Deleuze, Gilles. (1995) 2005. *Pure Immanence: Essays of a Life, Second Edition*. Translated by Anne Boyman. New York: Zone Books.
Derrida, Jacques. (1996) 1998. "For the Love of Lacan." In *Resistances of Psychoanalysis*, translated by Peggy Kamuf, Pascale-Anne Brault, and Michael Naas, 39–69. Stanford: Stanford University Press.
——. (2000) 2002. *Without Alibi*. Edited and Translated by Peggy Kamuf. Stanford, CA: Stanford University Press.
Glaberson, William. 2001. "Lawyers' Math in Sept. 11 Deaths Shows Varying Values for Life." *New York Times*, November 11. Available at: www.nytimes.com/2001/11/11/us/nation-challenged-lawsuits-lawyers-math-sept-11-deaths-shows-varying-values-for.html?module=Search&mabReward=relbias%3Aw. Last accessed July 20, 2014.
H.D. 1956. *Tribute to Freud: Writing on the Wall*. New York: New Directions.
Kamuf, Peggy. 2002. "Introduction: Event of Resistance." Introduction to *Without Alibi* by Jacques Derrida, translated by Peggy Kamuf, 1–27. Stanford: Stanford University Press.
Lacan, Jacques. (1959–1960) 1992. *The Seminar of Jacques Lacan, Book VII: The Ethics of Psychoanalysis 1959–1960*. Edited by Jacques-Alain Miller. Translated by Dennis Porter. New York: Norton.
Morris-Reich, Amos. 2002. "Simmel's and Lacan's Ethics of the Exception." *Telos* 123: 131–148.
Plato. 1982. *Phaedo*. Translated by R.S. Buck. Indianapolis: Bobbs-Merrill.
Rancière, Jacques. 2006. "Thinking Between Disciplines: An Aesthetics of Knowledge. *Parrhesia* 1 (1): 1–12.
Van Haute, Philippe. 2002. *Against Adaptation: Lacan's "Subversion" of the Subject*. New York: Other Press.
Wallace, David Foster. 2011. *The Pale King: An Unfinished Novel*. New York: Little, Brown and Company.

5 Death, Happiness, and the Meaning of Life—The View from Sociology

Introduction

The topic of death, often monopolized by theology, philosophy and even psychology through its studies of grief and bereavement, has rarely been treated as a signature of sociological theorizing except perhaps in empirical studies such as Durkheim's (1951) *Suicide.* Yet, in the sociological canon and particularly the classical works of Durkheim, Simmel, and Weber, a dialogical engagement with death as a collective representation is developed in ways often unstated and unthought. I want to make this engagement transparent as a discursive focus. I proceed by showing how the topos of death and its social character opens up inquiry in important ways, especially with respect to social relationships to meaning and what is called limit thinking. On this basis, I offer food for thought concerning the relationship between the treatment of death and (what Parsons called) "ultimate meaning" as topics on grounds of the charge that the morbidity of one (death) and the irresolute character of the other (ultimate meaning) can elicit only gratuitous fascination that needs to be put to rest as impractical, idle, antisocial or even subversive.

Form-giving Significance

> In every age, the cultivation of the innermost dimension of life interacts closely with the meaning it ascribes to death. How we perceive life and death are merely two aspects of a fundamentally unified attitude.
>
> (Simmel 2007, 73)

Georg Simmel sets upon this problem of the relationship between death and life and how it is represented as a collective representation. This means that he begins to frame the relationship to death as a problem in life, and as such, as a social phenomenon. Does death drive life or does life drive death from its precinct? Simmel's (2007) answer,

> [I]n every single moment of life we are those who must die, and each moment would be different if this were not in effect our predetermined condition. Just

as we are hardly already present at the moment of our birth, but rather something is continuously being born from us, so too do we hardly die only in our last moment.

(73)

"Form giving significance" is a way of saying that death drives life by inducing us to make something out of life, that the limitation that death brings to mind invites us to reflect upon how we make life matter or give it value. But this relation still seems contingent and intelligible in many ways unless we listen closely to Simmel's "form-giving significance." First, while Simmel is arguing for the place of death in life as a vital force not at all morbid, as having "form-giving significance," this awareness holds only for one attuned to such a relationship and to the need to keep it in mind throughout life in contrast to what Heraclitus called the sleepwalkers who push it aside. In contrast to these sleepwalkers, there are others whose only preoccupation in death is to avoid it, the survivors. Finally, there are those who treat death as modelled in the inert signifier or word, recognizing that this dead letter drives life, and so, that death is significant to life, but as an undifferentiated source of meaning-making, causing the social construction of value under its auspices. Simmel differs from sleepwalkers, survivors, and social constructionists in suggesting that death invests life with a desire for form and its discipline, and so, with an ideal (or ought) striving for more than survival, meaning-making or social construction, the desire to disclose in the diversity of life and its practices, the binding imperativeness of some sense of form in any situation of action, which means, some sense of the way in which the imaginary must be configured in social life for all actions and for friends and enemies alike.

Because Simmel (2010) grasps life as the Nothing in its primordial multiplicity in its being one thing as easily as any other, making Something out of Nothing reveals the connection between making and the Ought since any making needs to be guided by what it is that is being made. If death drives life insofar as the Ought (as the value of the need for collectedness) drives making, then death drives life to engage the form (Ought) imagined as binding the diversity of what is made.

The Ought takes shape both in driving social inquiry (the value assumed to ground inquiry in asking what is the value of inquiry) and in driving inquiry to work-through the material of the action studied (the value assumed to guide the content or commonplace in asking what is the value grounding sociability, composing a painting, a vase, gratitude, superordination). The Ought is a modernization of the Good in Plato. Death drives life to discern the power of the Ought through the message of the imaginary in any and all social phenomena. The imaginary is not the Good, but the theatre in which its variety and convoluted mixing and matching comes into play as our subject matter, the colliding manifestations of the Ought that we need a method to navigate, but a method that measures itself by respect for this play of the Ought. Death drives life insofar as it drives inquiry to submit to the Ought as guiding it and whatever it inquires into, subject and object becoming one in the folds of value, of the Ought. If the dead letter drives life as in the Lacanian formula, Simmel's embellishment says that the dead letter drives the need and desire to engage the Ought in any social endeavour, but always in ways that leave the relationship of the inquirer to the Ought as the uncertain legacy of the wide-awake subject of mortality. Thus, Simmel suggests that death drives life not simply in the way of making-meaning, but to accept the constraint of measuring words and deeds by respect for the continuation of a dialogical focus, and so, for some vision of shared being and of its remainder as fundamentally ambiguous.

In contrast to Weber and Durkheim, Simmel could have said, while it might be important for life to forget death in order to maintain its liveliness (to "bracket" it in some sense?), it is important not to forget that we forget (to do a turn from Derrida [2002] in another context). Simmel knows that in study and reflection upon the relations of life to death, such work is itself a way of negotiating that border and of affirming life through the art of a method of inquiry whose very topic in any study is the collision between form and life, and the question of whether and/or how the word is best brought to life. Any Simmelian analysis formulates the practice with an eye to the question of what conditions invest it with life essentially rather than externally, and how the collision between such conditions in the practice implicitly reflects the struggle in the narrative to make reference to the conditions that invest *it* (the analysis) with life essentially rather than externally. Here, Simmel treads a line that much inquiry would like to put to rest or exclude, much like death, the unspoken difference between what is essential and external. Is the risk of speaking at this border of meaning not analogous to the risk in any preoccupation with death? Yet, this is done as a way of working-through and developing a conversation over what kind of theorizing can resist deadening whatever it studies and what methods can be proposed for this.

Here, the problem of the relation of death to life is posed in the way of the human sciences, asking after the relation to death as a living practice in a manner that might and should activate sociology and psychoanalysis, among others. I want to begin to examine one part of such a discourse by asking how the material condition of death is represented in collective life as either/or (or neither/nor as Rancière says [see Blum, 2011b on either/ or v. neither/nor]; see Rancière, 1999, 2009, and its treatment in Blum, 2011b) to empower or undermine the desire that life is imagined as requiring.

The Secret of Life

Curiously, we owe to the sociologist Max Weber (1930) the key to the secret of life, from *The Protestant Ethic and the Spirit of Capitalism* where he said of capitalism "the problem is that of the Western bourgeoisie class and of its peculiarities" (p. xxxvii). Now if we think of capitalism as a figure of speech for the rut life inevitably falls into or follows, and of living a life as living in this manner and with these means as such, then something about the bourgeoisie should inform us about life and how to live it and alternatively could counsel us on the manner and means of morbidity (of death, the living death and how best to avoid it). Thus, Weber, the sociologist, might be offering us advice on how to be bourgeoisie where that can be understood as how to live life without permitting death to interfere, that is, how not to allow ourselves to be distracted by death. I think Weber is saying that though death is inevitable, it is the bourgeoisie who have mastered the art of concentrating upon life in a way free from that distraction. But then Simmel says that it is a vital part of the thoughtful life that thinks limits, to preserve the sense of death as an omnipresence in life.

Note how Lacan (1992, 303–304) creates a tension between happiness (which he identifies with the circulation of goods in the city) and death (which he identifies with thinking of limits). What is the relationship of happiness to death and how is the city factored into this relationship, or better, how does the materialism of the city dramatize the tension here?

> As I believe I have shown here in the sphere I have outlined for you this year, the function of desire must remain in a fundamental relationship to death. The question I ask is this: shouldn't the true termination of an analysis—and by that I mean the kind that prepares you to become an analyst—in the end confront the one who undergoes it with the reality of the human condition? It is precisely this, that in connection with anguish, Freud designated as the level at which its signal is produced, namely … distress, the state in which is that relationship to himself which is his own death … and can expect help from no one.

Lacan sets up death and our relationship to it in life as the locus of a discourse on happiness. Why should happiness be implicated in death unless we assume that the haunting of life by death (its undercurrent) compromises happiness? And yet if happiness is occasional, intermittent or even current, what is the relation of such a state to the thought of death? Better yet, how does (should, could) the thought of death influence life? Lacan (1992) offers the provocation as follows:

> Should the theoretical and practical purpose of our action be limited to the ideal of psychological harmonization? In the hope of allowing our patients to achieve the possibility of an untroubled happiness should we assume that the reduction of the antimony that Freud himself so powerfully articulated may be complete? I am referring to what he expresses in *Civilization and Its Discontents* when he affirms that the form in which the moral agency is concretely inscribed in man—and that is nothing less than rational according to him—the form he called the superego, operates according to an economy such that the more one sacrifices to it, the more it demands.
>
> (302)

Life then asks increasingly more of the one it seduced to desire, to need, and to lack:

> When in conformity with Freudian experience one has articulated the dialectic of demand, need and desire, is it fitting to reduce the success of an analysis to

> a situation of individual comfort linked to that well-founded and legitimate function we might call the service of goods? Private goods, family goods, domestic goods, other goods that solicit us, the goods of our trade or our profession, the goods of the city, etc. Can we, in fact, close off that city so easily nowadays? … To make oneself the guarantor of the possibility that a subject will in some way be able to find happiness even in analysis is a form of fraud.
>
> (Lacan 1992, 303)

Thinking at the limit is engaging the "distress" of one's finitude, that is, thinking in a way alive to one's death. This follows according to Simmel because the thought of death for the subject passing through a life creates the need and desire to reflect upon this passage as grounded in the way of a narrative with beginning and end, that always qualifies as a story about the passage that invariably is oriented to as a mark of value that distinguishes its bearer. The life and the Ought belong together insofar as the mortality of the passage drives their togetherness and need for discrimination. If death is disconcerting and in this way disturbs life and its aspiration to be comfortable with itself, then the thought of death as provocation becomes a theoretic strategy designed to subvert that very comfort which we can think of in this image of the city (collective life) as a circulation of goods, a circulation designed to produce a prosaic sense of "psychological harmonization" reflected in the notion of domestication. Then, the thought of death, properly aligned with the uncanny against domestication as if a sudden apparition, begins to point to the strange and queer sense of words and action, of life, when it is challenged by the thought of limit (Wittgenstein 1958; see also Blum 2003, 2011a, 2011b; Blum and McHugh 1984; Cavell 1979). It is as if these are countervailing forces, agonistic elements in the terrain of life, the city as the circulation of goods and over against this, the thought of limits, of death. Life then seems to have a secret automatism, as if a spell exercised upon us that keeps us working at it, the automatism we tend to capture in the formula of happiness and its chase:

> There's absolutely no reason why we should make ourselves the guarantors of the bourgeois dream. A little more rigor and firmness are required in our confrontation with the human condition … The establishment of the service of goods at a universal level does not in itself resolve the problem of the present relationship of each individual man to his desire in the short period of time between his birth and his death.
>
> (Lacan 1992, 303)

The "rigour and firmness required in our relation to the human condition" confirm that he does not renounce life or give up on life in his talk of death because he speaks for a relation in life, a living relation of rigour and firmness that has the desire to think limit, to think against the grain of the city in its domesticated shape as the circulation of goods. Theorizing as the thought of death can be nothing other than discipline or measured relations to civic speech and its formulaic distinctions, a way that demands and disciplines its talk precisely so as not to obey life mindlessly or reject it out of despair. Thus, happiness as a convention that could be otherwise, and is not to be celebrated or condemned mechanically, is a distinction, as formulaic as it is, that has to be engaged playfully and ironically in the guise of a theoretic actor who knows both its conventionality and its necessity as "equipment for living" (Burke, 1957) in the way of living distinctions that have a place in life at some time but could also be otherwise and otherwhere. So, if the bourgeoisie is a figure that represents the happy immersion in life and its pursuits, this allows us to understand Marx's cryptic comment on the proletariat, saying that they disclose the secret of capitalism. I suggest that he intends the proletariat to stand for the extinction of desire as a matter oriented to, as more of the same repetitively reinstated by life in its course. Their secret: the proletariat know that the bourgeoisie lie about life and death, acting as if there is no death; the proletariat know that life is more of the same, and that desire is never fulfilled except through dreamwork (see Blum 2003).[1]

Death and the Category

We see how sociology marks life by death in very important and generic ways when we examine the great founders, Durkheim, Weber, and Marx, each more or less accepting the notion that an investment in life requires a degree of unreason or irrationality due to the seductiveness of mortality itself and the hold of life upon the human subject. So Weber was struck by the irrational commitment to work as a surrogate form of salvation in the absence of any definitive reassurance about one's eternal life, making the commitment seem interesting to him by virtue of this very immersion in productive labor, as if a defence against the terrifying recognition of one's abandonment. Durkheim too imagined egoism as the natural lot of such a subject unless the social attachment, its complicated regimes of affiliation and expectation, could provide satisfaction strong enough to rectify separation. Both Weber and Durkheim view the fact of mortal life as potentially distracting in ways that need to be reimagined, reinvented, through what some might call fantasies about living on what we can think of after Kenneth Burke (1957) as "equipment for living" (I examine this conception of Kenneth Burke and develop an extended discussion of Weber's imaginary exchange with Tolstoy in Blum 2013, 253–262). The notion of life as an adjustment in this sense invites conceiving of the subject as reflective in an altogether different way, resisting what is known with some degree of zest and animation that might move with pleasure against the grain, that is, against itself, in ways that could appear self-destructive as if this is what life needs. While neither of these men took up the challenge of formulating the imaginary of such a modern subject, both identified the import of insistent drive in life as compelling.

Marx's notion of life as deadly was reflected in his division of the population into two classes as if a diversion (the "rat race") needed to distract them from apprehending the barren uniformity of social life that must invariably interrupt the collective sense of its natural equality. This notion of equality, of all humans as equal under the sign of mortality, at one and the same time makes of such a collective a horde fated to pass time until its death and immune to stimulation in the absence of anything for which to strive. In imagining these two classes, the haves and have-nots, he gave them each something to live for—accumulation, acquisition, holding on if lucky and aspiring to the same if unfortunate, imagining life as a game with winners and losers, allies and enemies, definite outcomes, rules and skills, plots and conspiracies, and bodies of know-how to be mastered in learning one's place and path.

In this way, if life needs to distract the human subject from death, everyone lives in accord with the illusion of stratification and by virtue of the need to learn about this illusion as such and to expose all to its dynamic. If self-worth is falsely tied to such an order (as if having and not having means what the order of stratification requires), then education must either be deceit or confrontation, with confrontation working to unsettle the illusion, and deceit simply seeking to pass it on. Marx tries desperately to make life satisfying for those who are tempted to treat it otherwise as if the repetitious reiteration of the same (Blum 2003). Thus, if Marx intuits how the bourgeoisie can continue living (their delusion about their self-worth prevents them from reflection, or makes them indifferent, which is the same), he poses the problem of how the proletariat can come to think of life as mattering, in the absence of the advantage of such distraction (and illusions) of the bourgeoisie.

Marx poses the problem of how one can live without illusion, not just pathetically or in resignation, but with a passion for life, trying to reinvent the imaginary of the proletariat as a *raison d'être* for living as such. In this gesture, as an unanticipated consequence of Marx's humanity, he also offers the emancipated segment of the bourgeoisie the opportunity to impersonate such an imaginary while remaining untouched as they are, as haves, by enabling them to think of themselves as proletariat, creating under the guise of critical thinking the delusional imaginary of liberalism as if a kind of cross-dressing. That is, if the lucky or opportune with advantage are to escape the burden of guilt, they need to imagine themselves as comparable to the proletariat (i.e. that knowing the truth of the lie gives them the kind of empathy that identifies them as the same, essentially). Similar in mind and not body, both classes are then fated to be the living dead, equal in that respect, equal by virtue of living without illusion. What Marx knows is that life cannot be endured without a fantasy, whether the imaginary of just deserts, of accumulation, inheritance and succession, or revolution, that life requires a belief in its mattering and that the two classes serve as a dramatic image of two shapes taken by such practices, as anomie (passing time, bourgeoisie) and toil (doing time, proletariat).

Classification

Durkheim's ambivalence towards death is reflected in different places and with often disparate implications (Durkheim 1933; see Blum 2013 for other examples). Durkheim redeems his indifference to the category or distinction (to the signifier) by showing how any category, in order to be meaningful, that is, to be alive and vital rather than dead, has to be made explicit and concrete as a social bond. Here is how he proceeds: any category, say, gender, age, race, Welsh, American, is abstract, undeveloped and implicit (empty in the idiom of Lacan) because the word (e.g. women) conveys an indivisibility that can only mask its internal diversification. The category is dead in the way any characterization is dead, announcing a unity supplied by the name and nothing more. In *Suicide*, Durkheim (1961, 180–202) proceeds by animating each category, imagining its diverse living conditions (thus, married or single women, urban or rural women, Protestant or Catholic women, women who work and women who do not) and in this way brings a category to life by enumerating the different ways in which it can be said to be attached to behavior. Yet, the list of variations seems to show that the category has no weight or force to collectivize the different ways it is done. Durkheim calls the social environment of such a category egoistic, existing only in and through its variations, as if all we might say about women or Americans (or about virtue as the "swarm of bees" in Plato's *Meno*) is that there are many kinds. This is the way of political economy according to Durkheim, the world of optimizing and transactions imagined between monadic, self-oriented agents (see Parsons 1949 for what must remain the best discussion).

Durkheim recognized in social life a countervailing tendency to arrest egoism through a stipulation of unity that invites loyalty and sacrifice at the expense of the diminution of voice. If Durkheim names such unity altruistic, it is for the reason that the sacrifice to the category occurs at the expense of the subject in ways that equate everyone by virtue of their being ruled by the same category as in a stereotype. Thus, the category has no weight when all women are treated as different and it has no weight when all women are treated as the same: such extremism in the deadly social environment does not nourish the mixed life in the relation of difference to unity. Therefore, if variation is at first necessary to animate the category, its unity must be redeemed and recovered in a way that is not stereotypical. Thus, in recognition of the importance of human variation for life, Durkheim shows the dangers of too much or too little as originating the desire for a mean position, making a reflective relationship to desire and its governance the sign of a healthy social life (and he goes further, suggesting that even a healthy environment is permeable and can become sick, forecasting in his way the impermanence of everything that comes to be).

So the category, like the statistic, is dead until animated by the capacity to imagine it as neither unregulated nor oppressive but as a relationship of limit to unlimited, of category to desire. For example, if the code limits the category of woman in the way grammar determines what we see, expect, name, and the like in relation to this regime, free individuals can still be inventive in relation to the code and the bond it both presupposes and implies. This is to say that being represented as man, woman, Welsh, American, is being identified as a subject of a symbolic order and as one necessarily subject to the inclusions, exclusions, rights, and relationships this order maintains (see Durkheim 1961, 297–325). At its best, the category operates as a social world in microcosm, binding, bonding, and orienting its subject in ways designed to depict a hold much stronger than a characteristic. Durkheim identifies this relationship of individuation to integration as the terrain of the symbolic order and of the ambiguous relation between the signifier (woman) and the process of signification through which it emerges. Thus, the category (woman, whatever) is only alive and vital when it is seen neither as a context for egocentrism nor for tyranny but as itself an object of desire as if a paradigm or standard of guidance. If life counteracts the living dead in any social environment, counteracts the altruistic and egoistic ties to life, then the speaker for vitality as a speaker for the category as a bond is the ideal speaker who orients to the category as if an ideal, as if what unifies the variety of women can only be the desire to make transparent the category as itself an object of desire. Thus, for any category, we can say that the ideal speaker is pro-life, must be conceived as that course of action that confirms the life of the category by rising above its externality in bringing it to view as if a standard of action. This is how we could say at the start of this exposition that Simmel had to formulate the relation of life to death as an ideal speaker.

This links the category to Benjamin's (1969) conception of the aura, for when Benjamin says of the relation that it originates in the primordial experience when "the person we look at or who feels he is being looked at, looks at us in turn" (akin to Parsons' double contingency). Similarly, if we invest the category (the word, the signifier, the inanimate mark) with "the ability to look back at us," we not only create a relationship (in a way that aesthetically can be said to do a neutralization of the commonplace by transforming it), but we also endow this lifeless "thing" with a capacity to rule us or hold us accountable in some sense by our looking up to it not as if it is punitive (aka: superego) but in accord with Lévinas' notion of the face that we see reflected in it as a sign of its openness to interpretation and vulnerability in that sense. In this experience of the aura, we bring the category to life, and if we revitalize our self in this gesture, it is only possible because we are prepared to see-as (see Blum 2011b, 37–38) in this way, that we desire of our self that we can rise to this occasion, investing the near-at-hand with this strange power to look back, to hold us accountable for its being seen, and in its way to make us "look up" by reminding us of something Other than other.

Like Durkheim, Max Weber treats death from the point of view of life in asking the question of the meaning of life, or what makes life worth living. Both Durkheim and Weber seem to imagine the subject as naturally drawn towards death but for an intervention that would help keep her alive. It is irrelevant that the intervention is the social tie in Durkheim and a dutiful commitment in Weber, because what collects them is that the intervention seems to both sociologists as if an irrational belief given the reality of human mortality. We could say that in this way sociology questions the self-evidence of life itself by finding it queer or odd in Wittgenstein's (1958) sense, odd that humans would keep on with life in the face of such inevitability.

More important, both say that this keeping at life is uncanny because it is not perfunctory or a matter of adapting with resignation to bad conditions, but devoted and enthusiastic to the point where it exceeds the expectations of these observers, that life and living is embraced in ways that can have important worldly results. Life then takes on a charged meaning when it seems to be lived at the edge of the border between living and dying, reminding us of Bataille's (1985, 116–130) formula for the general economy involving action guided by the expectation of loss as great as possible (war, gambling). Living at the edge (with an awareness of death in this sense) becomes the passion that enters into the overstimulated ambitious strivings both of anomie and of the energetic enterprising activities of commerce.

Whereas Durkheim more or less disregards the dynamics of this excess, anomie arising out of the desire to heal or reconcile the tension between the social and the personal, it seems that the instability of desire is a function of the continuous frustration aroused by unrealized satisfactions. That is, life must arouse desire that it cannot fulfil and can only displace in (what Lacan calls) frustration and aggression aroused by the desire of and for life, creating the constant alienation of the subject fated always to fall short of his or her own expectations. Durkheim's interlocutor could only be embodied as the stoic advice to limit one's expectations as a way of erasing the possibility of disappointment. Getting people to do more than is necessary is certainly the theme of Weber's *Protestant Ethic*, narrated as the progressive induction of the subject to embrace what is external (work) as a necessity, forcing him to elevate his interest in work by imagining it as the kind of activity his (and any) life requires to be meaningful.

Bourgeoisie: Life Affirmation and Flexibility

In Marx, the relation of bourgeoisie and proletariat reinstates this connection of life to death in showing how the death drive itself as life-affirmative and life-preservative depends upon contingencies not easily disregarded, such as poverty, but also misfortune and disease. Thus, the bourgeoisie personify that prized flexibility that the continuation of life requires of its subject. This means that obsolete objectives have to be redefined and not expurgated, have to be revised under the auspices of a rigorous notion of flexibility that takes the measure of "obsolete" attachments to metaphysics, recalculating them under the auspices of a new vision of communal accord in any present. But we must never forget how this great flexibility in self-development is exercised by foreclosing any and every thought of death.

The relentless revision of the relation to mortality in each present is empowered by what Weber noted as the link between inner isolation and the continuing need for proof of self-worth, the constant need for the reassurance of demonstrable productivity that remains the same even as its concrete conditions change. This is akin to the libidinal investment in self-love that Freud described in self-preservation and the need to repossess life, for example, as if life is the continuous rewriting of one's curriculum vitae. This suggests that the bourgeoisie, in part, express the life-affirming instinct of modernity everywhere by constantly inventing new ways of demonstrating one's self-worth to and for oneself and others, new gestures offering proof that we are not worthless in a world deserted by the assurance of salvation.

Thus, despite its historical associations with frugality and the expulsion of pleasure, asceticism animated by the desire of rigour is driven by the need and desire to be recognized as mastering the enjoyment of self-renunciation in an exemplary way, as one-of-a-kind, and so, as demonstrations or proofs of enjoyment in its guise as self-containment. What must then materialize is this tension inherent in the calculation of pleasure and it is the bourgeoisie of each generation that orchestrate this dialectical relation to the pleasure of productivity and the productivity of pleasure through the opportunity to question productivity itself. What the bourgeoisie know is that the ascetic displacement of pleasure in the service of the production of worldly accomplishments of enduring value requires for its persistence a continuous gesture affirming the mastery of self-renunciation as a spectacle exemplary for all who would wish to get on in such a world instead of languishing in dissatisfaction (in a way actually analogous to the pre-capitalist traditional resistances that Weber noted). The secret mastered here is that what must be renounced at any cost is the thought of death, and so, that what must be sacrificed is thought itself. That the sacrifice of thinking meaning is the cost life extracts makes this sacrifice the sign of good citizenship and its discipline and management a means of attaining pleasure.

Here, Weber concedes Marx's insight on the revolutionary character of the bourgeoisie, adding that this spiritual drive is reflected in their will to confront asceticism with the demands of emancipation in the service of constantly changing conceptions of pleasure. The bourgeoisie are particularly innovative with respect to pleasure, its creation and expansion, its social organization, and its dissemination. Weber's (1930) important recognition is that the productive life, fraught with anxiety because of the indeterminacy of the question of self-worth exacerbated by the withdrawal of the assurance of salvation, produces in its own way a dramatic sense of "inner isolation" as "a feeling of unprecedented inner loneliness of the single individual" (108). In this process, the risk of passion (living with the ambiguity of our commitments) is reconfigured by our readiness to freely will a methodical approach to the world so as to secure our place in ways undisturbed by the anxiety released through irresolute reflective conundrums. Inner loneliness as such is nothing other than the need to live life according to the death drive, to take pleasure in the unpleasure of "having" to live as an imperative to follow, to suffer, and to enjoy. Reflection redefines passion as the rigorous self-maintaining resolve required in any ambiguous situation. For example, today the notion of a career as an administrative project rather than vocation, and of the curriculum vitae as a constantly revised text as a prideful emblem of demonstrable productivity, is only the most prosaic indication of such redefined passion.

Proletariat: Fateful Life Chances, Resistance

When Marx says of the proletariat that they provide the (secret) key to understanding capitalism, he is pointing to their status as a figure for the extinction of desire that must limit the narcissism of life affirmation, though conceptions of "bare life" (Agamben 1998; see also Blum 1982 and 2011b, 125–166) give examples of extraordinary endurance in contrast to the capacity to rekindle life at any moment reflected in the perpetual motion and energetic activity of the bourgeoisie, stand besides the proletariat the compulsive inertia imagined of the living dead and of the aging, dying, diseased, and of the unlucky.

In therapy and education, the affirmation of life must be enforced as an objective for client, patient, student, that has to lead to the celebration of dialogue itself as the image of salvation that can rescue the subject from mortal destiny. That the belief in dialogue is equivalent to the belief in the affirmation of life must confirm any instance of resistance as morbid, that is, as defensive or uncooperative towards this common project. If analogues to such resistance show in silence, withdrawal, and the apathy of indolence and resignation, it can also be registered in resentment, cynicism, and the wordlessness that Baudrillard (1983) caricatured as the mass. In this sense, if death is always present in life as the interlocutor to the affirmative spirit of the drive to live in the shadow of its inevitability, as a reminder that this drive is a "detour" always haunted by the unspoken aura of life as if returning the look that knows the common fate, that knows the subject's detour is not immune to the path ahead, then the struggle to redeem conversation is part of the revolutionary impulse of the bourgeoisie. Understood thusly, revolutionizing the mass, the client, patient, student or whatever, amounts to revitalizing life affirmation always under the shadow of the sneer and the taunt or, more strongly, the silence that haunts life. The detour itself invites this silence to punctuate and penetrate verbosity in ways that can only distinguish the volubility of the bourgeoisie from reflective speech (as we are trying so hard to do here for death and its place in life). Note the dialogue between art and nihilism in the novels of Elena Ferrante (2012) on Naples (particularly *My Brilliant Friend*, translated from the Italian by Ann Goldstein).

The Modernization of Enlightenment

The sociological approach suggests that whether or not a reflection upon death is part of a thoughtful life is revealed less through fixation upon the meaning, content or significance of death per se, but to the ways in which representations of death are managed, handled or negotiated in collective life. What I call modernization of enlightenment serves to rescue theorizing from an impossible engagement with ambiguity in a gesture of renunciation that will still have costs. Note Stanley Cavell's (1988) formulation of Kant:

> You can take these paragraphs as constituting the whole argument of the *Critique of Pure Reason*, in four or five lines: (1) Experience is constituted by appearances. (2) Appearances are of something else, which cannot itself appear. (3) All and only functions of experience can be known; these are our categories of the understanding. (4) It follows that the something else—that of which appearances are appearances, whose existence we must grant—cannot be known … (5) Moreover, since it is unavoidable for our reason to be

> drawn to think about this unknowable ground of appearance, reason reveals itself to itself in this necessity also.
>
> (30)

If practical thinking elects to forgo this "something else" as unknowable, it still recoups its strength through such a limitation. Although we are frequently "drawn" to think about this "unknowable ground of appearance," and so, must struggle with such a temptation (in a way that is passionate), to give in is impetuous, inviting us to understand our best interests to lie in our power to *will* our freedom from such a "necessity" in order to escape from the inevitability of such temptation (and all of its "imaginary" convolutions and antinomies).

In this sense, the imaginative structure of the Enlightenment includes renunciation insofar as, in the way of Kant, it accepts the idea that we can at best know only appearances but not the in-itself, making the desire for the in-itself *under such conditions* impetuous and self-destructive. In this way, the enlightened affirmation of freedom that Kant celebrates is ascetic at its core, a gesture that must renounce passionate striving for the in-itself, the desire to express the "inexpressible," on the ground that such renunciation is a primary expression of our freedom (we *could* after all remain superstitious, freely allowing ourselves to be determined by false idols, in submitting to the charm of being driven in such ways).

If the secret known by the bourgeoisie as I have discussed is the mastery of self- management reflected in the renunciation of thinking the limits, this secret is not simply a fragment of "know-how" but backed up and justified by a notion of public spiritedness that not only makes it a commitment good in itself but treats its denial as evil. This commitment can be first grasped in a rudimentary way in the idea of the necessity of being practical not in the sense of mercenary, utilitarian, hard-hearted but as concerns attentive to practical situations in life that seem relatively intractable, much as in the Confucian notion of practicality as a willingness to "let it be."

Here, the practical actor is formulated not simply as a business person but as one who is attentive and disciplined towards sustaining and maintaining the body and presumably life, not out of an interest in survival as an end in itself, but as means for furthering other aims. If such care and circumspection (in Heidegger's lingo) is good, its contrast, whether viewed as romantic, self-indulgent or capricious, is condemned.

David Bates (2001) captures dramatically the political implications of the ban on ambiguity among enlightenment thinkers, who were simultaneously aware of the "truth" of ambiguity as such and at the same time oriented to the need to disavow it in practice:

> There was then no doubt that any exploration of the unknown was still a radical risk. Hobbes actually explained why with great clarity. Truth and falsity, he said, are in speech alone, in human forms of knowledge. We can try to eliminate falsity by seeking out the irrational or incoherent connections within our own thought. But we should remember, he said, that these human

> truths purged of ambiguity were only contingent certainties, because we can never be entirely sure what we might encounter in the future… . Similarly in Jean-Jacques Rousseau's *Social Contract*, the body of citizens may fail to find the sublime truth of the general will in its laws; however the one who actively disrupts the established order, the one who willingly breaks the law, must be put to death (or exiled).
>
> (8)

In other words, error is endemic; the Grey Zone is inescapable because of the omnipresence of ambiguity (See Locke, 1690). Such knowledge enjoins us to forfeit as the wrong way, as a criminal or antisocial path, what cannot be limited or determined. Bates (2001) describes how Turgot, the abbe Sieyes and others condemned "metaphorical straying" as antisocial by distinguishing between the "normal" human fallibility of the citizen and the oriented pursuit of meaning by the criminal: "So for Robespierre, the errancy of the patriot had to be distinguished from the criminal deviation of the enemy," marking a difference between error and crime that could convert the error of fallibility into the virtue of "being practical" in contrast to the resistance shown (18). Note that this distinction between the right and wrong path, error and crime, and citizen and criminal differs from the decisive fork in the road enunciated by Parmenides as the contrast to the way of seeming and the way of becoming, or Heraclitus' being all ears and attuned to the logos in contrast to being a sleepwalker: in the modernization of this fork in the road, the one who is on the wrong road travels knowingly out of a belief that it is necessary and desirable for life.

Conclusion

The undiscussed engagement with the question of mortality and the relationship to death in life is recovered through a reading of the classics of sociology—Durkheim, Marx, Simmel, and Weber—and the works of Freud and Lacan, to dramatize the relationship of such a concern to the imaginary of perpetual happiness idealized by the bourgeoisie of each generation and exemplified as the "problem" of the city.[2] If engaging mortality is conceived as an example of the thinking of limits, it is proposed that this ban parallels disavowing the question of meaning that the bourgeoisie have cultivated and perfected in the name of practical thinking. In this way, the bourgeoisie can be said to have mastered the secret of life and the connection between mental hygiene and intellectual parsimony celebrated by Kant as the advance of enlightenment. In this sense, the conditions of citizenship in the city are said to require a systemic disregard of such "deep" concerns on Kantian grounds that their inaccessibility and irresolute character can only distract circumspection from its limited goals. Yet, the imaginary relationship in life cannot be extinguished, making the relationship to the unknown, its ambiguity and remainder, intractable and fertile, occasioning the range of situations we study and inhabit. If the bourgeoisie are correct that a phobic preoccupation with death is distracting to life just as a phobic and phallic obsession with meaning destroys the poetry of thought, we know that forgetting death, like forgetting meaning, is complex enough to require not an either– or relationship but the forgetting that is capable of remembering what it lays aside, not amnesia, disavowal or repression, but something akin to the absolute humour that Baudelaire (1983) describes as acting as if it is ignorant of what it really knows. Although I have not discussed Simmel's marginalization during his life in any way here, I have hinted ever-so slightly that his solution to the anxiety of death and to the anxiety of ultimate meaning should begin to make reference to the price he might have paid for this and to this debt that we will work to redeem for him now and in the future.

Notes

1 The relation of life to death, or the question of how life and the living should handle death, was given primordial expression as a "problem" in the discourses of Stoicism and Epicureanism in classical Greece.

2 It might be said that the conditions affecting death and its representation today have changed because of the influences of biomedicine, but I have suggested that this seems simply an extension of the foreclosure of meaning of the bourgeoisie and its molecular idealism that hopes to outwit mortality (Blum 2012, Blum 2013).

References

Agamben, Giorgio. (1982) 2006. *Language and Death: The Place of Negativity*. Translated by Karen E. Pinkus and Michael Hardt. Minneapolis: University of Minnesota Press.

Bataille, Georges. (1933) 1985. "The Notion of Expenditure." In *Visions of Excess: Selected Writings 1927–1939*, edited by A Stoekl, translated by Allan Stoekel and Donald M. Leslie Jr, 116–130. Minneapolis, MN: University of Minnesota Press.

Bates, David. 2001. "Idols and Insight: Enlightenment Topography of Knowledge." *Representations* 73 (1): 1–23.

Baudrillard, Jean. (1977 and 1981) 1983. *Simulations*. Edited by Sylvère Lotringer. Translated by Paul Foss, Paul Patton, and Phil Beitchman. New York: Semiotexte.

Benjamin, Walter. (1936) 1969. "The Work of Art in the Age of Mechanical Reproduction." In *Illuminations: Essays and Reflection,* edited by Hannah Arendt, translated by Harry Zohn. New York: Schocken Books, 217–252.

Blum, Alan. 1982. "Steps in the Self Understanding of the Experience of Suffering an Affliction: Victim, Patient, Client, Pariah. Reflections" *Canadian Journal of Visual Impairment* 1: 64–82.

——. 2003. *The Imaginative Structure of the City*. Montreal: McGill-Queen's University Press.

——. 2011a. *The Grey Zone of Health and Illness*. Bristol: Intellect Press.

——. 2011b. "Life, Death and the In-Between: The Duck/Rabbit and the Face of the Clown." In *Spectacular Death: Interdisciplinary Perspectives on Mortality and (Un) representability*, edited by Tristanne Connolly, 21–41. Bristol: Intellect Press.

——. 2013. "Durkheim's Ruse: The Concept as Seduction." *Canadian Journal of Sociology* 39 (4): 567–594.

——. 2014. "Guide for the Perplexed: Science and Literature as Equipment for Living (In Preparation)." *Philosophy and Rhetoric* 48 (1): 54–72.

Blum, Alan and Peter McHugh. 1984. *Self-Reflection in the Arts and Sciences*. Atlantic Highlands, NJ: Humanities Press.

Burke, Kenneth. 1957. *The Philosophy of Literary Form: Studies in Symbolic Action.* Berkeley, CA: University of California Press.

Cavell, Stanley. 1979. *The Claim of Reason: Wittgenstein, Skepticism, Morality, and Tragedy*. Oxford: Oxford University Press.

——. 1988. *In Quest of the Ordinary: Lines of Skepticism and Romanticism*. Chicago, IL: University of Chicago Press.

Derrida, Jacques. (2000) 2002. *Without Alibi*. Edited and Translated by Peggy Kamuf. Stanford, CA: Stanford University Press.

Durkheim, Émile. (1893) 1933. *The Division of Labor in Society*. Translated by George Simpson. New York: The Free Press.

——. (1912) 1961. *The Elementary Forms of the Religious Life*. Translated by Joseph Ward Swain. New York: Collier Books.

——. 1951. *Suicide: A Study in Sociology.* Edited by George Simpson. Translated by John A. Spaulding and George Simpson. New York: Glencoe.

Ferrante, Elena. 2012. *My Brilliant Friend.* Translated by Ann Goldstein. New York: Europa Editions.

Lacan, Jacques. (1959–1960) 1992. *The Seminar of Jacques Lacan, Book VII: The Ethics of Psychoanalysis 1959–1960*. Edited by Jacques-Alain Miller. Translated by Dennis Porter. New York: Norton.

Locke, John. 1690. *An Essay Concerning Human Understanding*. Available at Project Gutenberg: www.guten- berg.org/browse/authors/l#a2447

Parsons, Talcott. 1949. *The Structure of Social Action.* Glencoe, IL: The Free Press.

Rancière, Jacques. (1995) 1999. *Disagreement: Politics and Philosophy*. Translated by Julie Rose. Minneapolis: University of Minnesota Press.

——. 2009. *The Emancipated Spectator*. Translated by Gregory Elliott. London: Verso.

Simmel, Georg. (1910) 2007. "The Metaphysics of Death." Translated by Ulrich Teucher and Thomas M. Kemple. *Theory, Culture & Society* 24 (7/8): 72–77.

——. (1918) 2010. *The View of Life: Four Metaphysical Essays with Journal Aphorisms*. Translated by John A.Y. Andrews and Donald N. Levine. Chicago: University of Chicago Press.

Weber, Max. (1905) 1930. *The Protestant Ethic and the Spirit of Capitalism*. Translated by Talcott Parsons. London: George Allen & Unwin.

Wittgenstein, Ludwig. (1953) 1958. *Philosophical Investigations*. Edited by G.E.M. Anscombe and R. Rhees. Translated by G.E.M. Anscombe. New York: Macmillan.

6 Ending and Beginning

Introduction

The last chapter proposed that thinking of mortality represents in an important sense something like a prohibition in social life not simply because it is denied out of fear in the so-called denial of death model but for the reason that such a thought, if recurrent, is a dangerous preoccupation that can interfere with commitment to the meaningfulness of the present at any time. We noted that if the recurrence of such a thought is difficult to manage and an impediment to the administration of jouissance, it can also enlist in its cause, a view of its subversive character because of its temptation to challenge conventional thought by its focus upon the inscrutable limits of life and meaning. In this chapter I begin to examine the ways in which this fascination can pervade and unsettle conduct in everyday life.

Dying and Death

The difference between dying and death is significant insofar as the life of dying tends to be treated as the limited case of the notion whereas we have suggested that the life of dying at its best (and worst) could orient to the unthinkability of death in ways that make this impasse (whether to accept or deny such an intellectual force) the sign of the reflective border in living. That is, at its best life must think about death rather than dying if it is the thought of death that gives form to our life. If the thought of death is absorbed by the anticipation of the experience of dying, this empirical relation to mortality limits the subject while at the same time, repressing anxiety until the last moment by refusing to think past the destination of the dying body. The constant threat of the thought of death to break through this foreclosure creates the phenomenon of one's falling apart and makes the life being lived at this point (the point of the traumatic recognition) a life ruled by the anticipation of eternity and its monadic self-understanding as destiny.

Dying is a lived experience and in a sense it begins as long noted, with birth, since finitude is the name of the game and as the cliché says, living is preparation for death, our common destination. If it is obvious in this sense that the living body is the dying body, this equivalence still cannot provide for the distinctiveness of the dying body as part of life, making the cliché banal or at best, empty. So how can we appreciate the lived experience of the dying body without seeing it on the one hand as more of life and on the other hand, as say, sickness? Or how can we see the experience of dying as something more than aging and something more than deterioration but as an orientation to an order?

Here are the choices: either living as dying is equivalent to aging which we can consider a formless notion since it gives the life of dying no specific form, or it is linked to decline, deterioration, and/or to surviving in ways that make it seem only negative deprivation and/or compensatory as in holding on to what one has or is trying to regain. Thus, to conceive of the social form of dying as, paradoxically, full of life, as a living and specific course of action, we have to resist identifying this orientation with experience per se as a connection too generic such as simply aging, or on the other hand with bare life, or with the experience of illness, all of these ideas focusing on usages either as too general on the one hand or on the other as too extreme. We can ask then, what is the form of the life of dying if the lived experience of the dying body is not simply the reverse of the experience of life and vitality (say, of the child and such innocence and engagement), nor of the resigned demoralization of bare life (say, of captivity), or of sickness (say, chronic disease)?

Note that what we are resisting here are cultural stereotypes that remain part of the collective discourse on the lived experience of the dying body, whether as the simple process of aging defined tautologically as the course of a mortal life, or an experience of resigned captivity, or of chronic disease that is dominated in this way by an overriding sense of loss. It is important to see that these views of the dying body can influence care for such persons. In other words, such views influence us to see mortality itself and its evolutionary self-understanding as decline. The often imputed childishness of the aged seen as correlative to a kind of helplessness and withdrawal is mixed with the recognition that the innocence and vitality of childhood is lost for those who age, and not only for the aged but for any adults as such. Thus, sentimentality over lost childhood is a constant theme and focus of nostalgia in collective life. If innocence is supposed to be eroded by aging, its loss produces a kind of sentimentality that we might conceptualize as related to melancholia or mourning for the desolation inflicted by abandonment. On the other hand, if aging is seen as captivity or as illness and decline, then provisioning, tolerance, and nurturance are typically viewed as the only adequate responses to such resignation and dependency. The intimate is seen as suffering aging and is typically treated either as increasingly childlike, while lacking the resources of such energy and capacities, or as an inmate or patient. Note that the inevitability of this view of aging as a condition, summons it to mind as a common fate that enables the one who cares, to view the subject as a mirror of shared being, a portent of what he or she will also come to, that is, as a reflection of what one and all are fated to undergo at some point, revealing in this way that both the one who cares and the one cared for are united by this condition that happens only in the present to differentiate one from the other at this time but not fundamentally, disclosing in its way a universal passage (see Blum 2013). Yet, because the universality of this passage tends to be overwhelmed by the force of the present and its inescapable totality, there seems to be nothing other than what is present to us in the present.

Inevitability

Here then, we have a sense of togetherness produced by this idea of shared being (that we all have a common destination), registered in a truism that cannot do more than amuse us. Note that the cliché that no one can die for another counteracts this sense of a uniform destination by its intimation of our inviolable separateness from these others. This difference, as a phenomenological event, was the theme of Georg Simmel's work. Despite the shared inevitability of death, the lived experience of the body seems to distinguish us as if the experience of dying is intimate in some sense and the inevitability of death as an unknown finality discloses the anonymity at the core of our commonness because of the way this apprehension of death seems to belong to each alone as specific and incomparable. It is as if when we think of our common death we tend to formulate our self as part of a condition in which our participation is relative to the others, whereas when we orient to the life of dying it appears to be an absolute and singular apprehension that is closed in its particular way to all but oneself.

Simmel constantly emphasizes the tension between the experience of togetherness and apartness, that our sense of being reduced to the common and species being is necessarily undermined by our need to absolutize ourselves as unique, experiencing our self as part of a totality (i.e. society) and as a totality in itself (individuality). Simmel then reformulates the "tragedy" of life not simply in terms of the contrast between the social (as normative) and the individual, but as a collision between life and form that is registered in the idea of the Grey Zone of life and death, that life dies and dying lives in one and the same moment. Many have remarked on this contrast as if in one case we think of ourselves as a vital and sovereign being and in the other case as a thing relative to all of the other items of nature that meet a common end (Lacan's das Ding, Bataille's intimate and thing, finite and infinite etc.). For example, in speaking of the tension between the individual and society, Simmel reminds us that even if we affirm that "society" is a social construction, that it is nothing but a sign.

> We must still admit the existence of conflict between the two. One reason… is the fact that, in the individuals themselves, social elements fuse into the particular phenomenon called "society." "Society" develops its own vehicles and organs by whose claims and commands the individual is confronted as by an alien party. A second reason results from another aspect of the inherency of society in the individual. For man has the capacity to decompose himself into parts and to feel any one of these as his proper self. Yet each part may collide with any other and may struggle for the dominion over the individual's actions. This capacity places man … into an often contradictory relation with those among his impulses and interests that are not preempted by his social character. In other words, the conflict between society and

> individual is continued in the individual himself as the conflict among his component parts.
>
> (Simmel 1955, 59)

That is, the conflict among values is "played out" within language itself in a way that typifies any collective as the scene of such concerted play.

In this way, I want to identify the ambiguity not simply as the tension between individual and society but in the condition of mortal existence that discloses how the inevitability of our common condition and fate in death is made unique and singular (absolute, intimate) because of our memory that stimulates images that will expire with us, revealing how our loss of life is simultaneously an anticipation of the loss of the positioning of others for us and in us as part of who we are to ourselves, the intimacy we register as our being present to our presence at present, disclosing that our death is in its way a reiteration of their death since they live after only with us. Our dying risks inflicting upon those who have been part of us, a second death, unless we are able to perpetuate them through the remains of images to others, at best in the varied representations and influences that we might be lucky enough to leave for others after, if we are fortunate enough to be remembered by such others in the face of their short-lived energies, interests, and affections.

What seems like a narcissistic dream of self-extension here might just be the way the dying body is exercised by memory as work in the present for the social being as custodian of an intimate archive. This lived experience of dying suggests that with the expiration of the body, the remains of all the moments "belonging" to the person jointly and its body, risk perishing. If every death threatens history in this way, a dying subject (not simply as captive, sick, or aging) can be expected to know and be exercised by this condition, and to desire to put it into words for others. The putting into words that such self-extension signals is then not simply like a boast or obituary that records personal achievements but seems similar to an archive of moments and what Simmel calls the adventures that add up to the self as a person.

Indeed, Freud made reference to the self as an archive of sorts with its many and diverse files. Perhaps the drive to transmit such an archive accounts both for the ramblings of dementia and the obsessively sentimental tales of the loquacious reconstructions of the aging subject who relentlessly passes on versions of the past that seem special and noteworthy. We might say that this difference long noted between the person as intimate and as a thing is registered in the difference between story and record. The life of the dying body can then be said to dwell at this border, contemplating how such a difference might end in after life with the expiration of the body. Thus, the specter of inevitability reminds us that we who are bound and bonded together in mortality must experience anonymity in relation to one another and to our common prospects that are unknown, dramatizing for us each in any present a kind of basic equality that was effaced in life and remains oblique but true. Yet, such inevitability and the equality it might summon to mind can only invite us to dwell upon the intimate and singular history that we inherit and desire to reveal and to pass on as what remains.

Intimacy

Our intimacy is not simply an unproblematic and undivided assortment of images that can be said to belong to us, but serves as grounds for inference and diagnosis of what and who we were and are. The diagnosis stands to the archive that informs it as the self-knowledge that symptoms can only intimate. Where is the location of the "Me" (rather than the "I") and the "who" (rather than the "what") in the flux passing as the external images and relationships that appear to be mine? The demand to connect and to attempt reconnecting the external to the intimate whether for the self (the symptom, unconscious, interest, motive), the other (the other person, mind, recognition), nature (the environment), and the word (sign, signifier) persists as the ineluctable and incurable scene of ambiguity that can endure as the demand that haunts the life of the dying body. We can question this in different ways: just where am I in all of this "stuff?" Or, what in this debris of moments and attachments can be said to belong to me essentially rather than externally?

We say that intimacy as some sense of being in proximity to our self, being close to our self in the special way of irreconcilable singularity (even if a phonocentric illusion), confers this authority upon us by virtue of its secrecy and the covert succession of discrete and unshared moments about which one might have (borrowing from Everett Hughes) guilty knowledge, or better as in Simmel, some sense of the very special erotic turning points that mark a life and its adventures, that succession of opportunities both taken and missed that become vestigial pieces of our archive.

This distinction we have noted throughout between absolutism and relativism, my death for me and for other, as we suggest, resonates with Simmel's conception of the difference between the individual as a whole (absolutism) and as a part (relativism) but is grounded in Plato's notion of the relation of Same and Other: for example, as the Same the individual is a part similar to all of the other parts, and as Other is differentiated and autonomous in relation to the other parts. In needing to resist the either/or of the extremes of relativism or absolutism the individual resists the idea that one's death is the death of the world. In terms of our method of engaging social conduct we observe the relationship between Same and Other in any practice and with respect to any signifier when we recognize it (see it as) to be dealing with the problem of the tension between Same and Other, for example, just as the convention or signifier enforces a sameness upon us, it also requires the differences elicited by our orienting to it and interpreting it. In contrast, the best example of indifference to this impasse is seen in the logic of the total institution whether the asylum or concentration camp, bureaucracy, or the standardization of quantification, big data and the like, all viewing their requirement of organizing and controlling a population as an exigency forcing them to see the world as dead.

Even when death is represented, for example in mass media, we can say that the world is not kept alive in the stories that reject theorizing death on any level for the presentation of visuals that simply show death as a façade or horrific event without rhyme or reason. Such visuals show life as interrupted by death as a kind of random event presented in the absence of reflection instead of using death as a provocation to elicit meaning. If the suicide bomber and terrorism are animated by the idea that people are only engaged by what they see without reflecting upon anything but the horror and externality of an accident, capitalist media simply show the horror of scenes of death without explanation (except simple-minded frustration-aggression accounts). In these ways what Simmel calls the form-giving significance of death is quieted except in the interruptions of war, terror, crime, legal judgment, or atrocity that can function to make death a spectacle rather than an occasion for reflection, also in the lamentation of the old and their intimates that always risk banality.

Maturity

When at its best, age is treated as akin to maturity, this empirical conception of the subject typically makes its strength depend upon its capacity to learn from experience (and the cliché that history is informative) in order to apply the lessons of longevity to its present. In contrast, I suggest that age permits us to use maturity as a robust notion, not simply as equivalent to experience, but as a way of rethinking what a reflective relationship to chronology might assume, other than sagacity at best and cynicism at worst (Blum 2013). Here, we might appreciate the lesson of maturity to be closer to the capacity for tact that Gadamer discussed as part of an ability to navigate the border between anonymity and intimacy. That is, the anonymity of language and its automated classifications, assumptions, interdictions, and grammatically legislated moves and positions is always challenged by the desire to usurp the sanctity of linguistic conventions in order to restore the intimacy of the signifier. Just as this tension between anonymity and intimacy haunts language as a border, so does it inhabit the speaker's relation to the self as an innermost enigma, say in the puzzle of self-knowledge, striving for some kind of reconciliation between the self as a thing (say, a body) and its intimate register (Blum 2014; Blum 2015). The example of aging typically makes this border a problem for its subject. Yet, as Simmel shows, we do not require the example of aging to appreciate the ambiguity of such a border since any social interaction dramatizes to us this "gap" between intimacy and anonymity in the recognition that we can never know the other person completely:

> One can never know another person absolutely, which would involve knowledge of every single thought and mood. Nevertheless, one forms some personal unity out of those of his fragments in which he alone is accessible to us. This unity, therefore, depends upon the portion of him, which our standpoint permits us to see.
>
> (Simmel 1950, 308)

If maturity in some way begins to address the problem of self-knowledge for the subject of aging, we note further that maturity is often contrasted with infantilism or childishness. Assuming the contrast not to be intended developmentally in the most prosaic way, we might revive the connection of infantilism and childishness as a positive relationship, say to innocence, which allows us to consider maturity as a way of handling its loss. In this way, we can imagine a situation of action for aging as the problem of producing in some way an engagement with the demand for innocence to be constantly revised and revived at different points in the passage of life. If anonymity makes reference to our sharing this loss of innocence, intimacy would begin to speak to how we translate such loss (or "handicap") into a virtue.

Kenneth Burke (1957, 16) called such conditions (even finitude) handicaps, suggesting that part of the ingenuity, inventiveness, and creativity of any engagement is to translate this handicap or burden into an incentive. Burke says in this respect that "a threat is the basis of beauty" in the way the "puzzle of mortality and its burden appears enigmatic" (see Blum, 2011a, 52). Following Tiffany (ibid.) I suggested that "analogous to the spellbinding character of the riddle" that he noted after Adorno, "is the fascination exercised by the burdens of health and the threat of death." As I am using it, the threat raised by death is the threat of the loss of our life and the enigma of its meaning for our action in the present.

> The metaphor of the philistine towards the obscurity of the poem that establishes the form of modern art and the desire of the subject to pursue the meaning of the poem is the archetype for the ideal speaker that keeps life alive, keeps death at bay, through the dialogical engagement with the enigma and its obscurity. This is to say … that it is the … enigma of self-knowledge that keeps death at bay in ways that can only occur when the enigma is seen as a riddle with potential, disclosing obscurity as incentive for the animation of desire rather than the promise of annihilation. The question of desire then becomes one of seeing obscurity as stimulating and life-affirming (as puzzle or riddle) rather than as deadly.
>
> (ibid.)

Now we can begin to hear intimacy and the sovereignty it presupposes as its conceit to mark the loneliness that Dumm (2008) identifies as a pervasive dimension of the condition of the human subject through the registers of solitude in loss, love, and grieving. If Freud (1957) says of such solitude that it depends upon a narcissistic object choice, this should not simply be disavowed as if false consciousness, as the "humanist" illusion of sovereignty, but analyzed as part of the work of the imaginary and its convoluted configurations.

The Discursive Façade of Intimacy: Hallucinating as Social Action

It is important to reintroduce Bataille at this point in order to expand the discussion of the subject. Such a subject strives to imagine the self (oneself) intimately rather than reductively. This was the question Georges Bataille (1989, 50–52) took upon himself to suffer in writing.

> Intimacy cannot be expressed discursively… . What is intimate in the strong sense, is what has the passion of an absence of individuality … I will resort to articulation nevertheless… . The separate individual is of the same nature as the thing, rather the anxiousness to remain personally alive that establishes the person's individuality is linked to the integration of existence into the world of things… . He would have no anguish if he were not the individual (the thing), and it is essentially the fact of being an individual that fuels his anguish. It is in order to satisfy the demands of the thing, it is insofar as the world of things has posited his duration as the basic condition of his worth that he learns anguish. He is afraid of death as soon as he enters the system of projects that is the order of things. Death disturbs the order of things and the order of things holds us. Man is afraid of the intimate order that is not reconcilable with the order of things.

The intimate order, in this case as the unspoken desire for the eternality of the present and of my presence (see Blum 2008) makes reference to what can be thought but not spoken, the surfeit that seems to exceed determination. For the caregiver too, whether witness or intimate, the problem remains one of orienting to the subject as engaged by this question and its need to be situated with respect to the range of other conditions that are correlative with the passage. So if the sufferer is seen as trying to grasp herself intimately rather than as a thing, the caregiver can be viewed as trying to grasp the sufferer intimately rather than as a thing.

Thus the incommunicable intimate order must necessarily be glossed by any vision of the correlation of aging with physical deterioration because this order, reflecting the history of a person, must exceed as "infinitely more" a chronological conception of the person as an entity measured by a record of external milestones.

Here in the moment of the present between past and future, we conceive of a subject orienting to the unknown in two senses, with respect to what one will come to and what will be made of one in the face of what is not yet, and how what is both lost and retained in one's past can and must come to pass as inaccessible for those who will follow. Thus, the intimate character of the experiences we retain, dissolve with us even though we have and might continue to represent them for another, and so in this way are marked by them as singular just as much as the events they are meant to recall. Those events, lost to any other but us, are destined to be lost to all because they are only ours and what is ours will be lost forever more. The inevitability of the loss of what is mine and what "belongs" to me is the very condition of my singularity that seems to absolutize me to and for myself as what I am and what is irretrievable by any other. That this intimate archive cannot be guarded and preserved through time is a function of singularity that must suffer the same fate. In fact singularity can be nothing other than this sense of the inevitable disappearance of who I am to myself in just this sense. The gap between the witnessing that might testify to and for us, and what I have that can never be known as such and is lost to them, can only be anticipated for them as a vestige of what I have, perhaps recycled as their intimate archive also destined to be lost to whosoever witnesses for them. Make no mistake: though death does not necessarily take me out of circulation as a sometimes-trace, it spells the end for me of what I have and hold, what I am to and for myself alone, here and now. The mental anguish of the aged might just refer to the need to disengage from such a thought, to let it rest in peace in this present.

Putting into Words

On this ground I want to open up a path for interrogating the action of hallucinating as a way of speaking allegorically about other matters that the subject at end-of-life is exercised by and attempts to articulate, as a method for making reference to the anxiety and phenomenon of "putting into words" as a necessary and unfulfillable task.

I try to intervene in this discourse not by treating it as ideological or distorted but as idiomatic in its desire to construct a world by representing what cannot be put into words, in reaching into the unknown by anticipating a future that might receive its work. In this sense the hallucination as dream happens in the future in the time of its interpretation and (Marder 2013, 210) overcomes anxiety because the subject is not alone but co-present with the future that will receive it. This is how the strong sense of a future that will receive our influence remains essential to the lived experience of the subject and its extinction by whatever means can only produce fear and trembling. It is in this sense that an end has to imagine itself as a beginning.

The aged know in this sense that time reveals sovereignty as the conceit of singularity, singularity driven to need and desire to misrecognize its autonomy and "personhood" as eternal and transient, as its feint of absolutism, as its gesture of absolute humor (see my use of Baudelaire in Blum, 2011b, 25–38) as if unaware of what it knows here, as both necessary equipment for living *and* necessarily irretrievable for eternity. In bringing to the surface the recognition that death itself (really temporality) is both relative and absolute, finite and infinitely more, aging can (in the strongest sense) recognize the essential paradox of life in time, of what Baudelaire (1972) calls the coexistence of the temporal and the eternal as the condition of the present that needs to be engaged.

Thus, in its way, the inducement of life to believe in it and commit with verve to its hold and consequentiality can become problematic in ways that can make the end-of-life itself an enigma *at* the end-of-life. Recall again how Bataille (1989, 47) dramatizes this hyperbolically.

> The power of death signifies that this real world can only have a neutral image of life, that life's intimacy does not reveal its dazzling consumption until the moment it gives out. No one knew it was there when it was; it was overlooked in favour of real things, death now one real thing among others. But death suddenly shows that the real society was lying.

In other words, life demands that we push death aside, laying it to rest as simply one fact among many; but end-of-life can begin to expose this ban as a lie, disclosing in its way that death was the only fact worth considering, making the end-of-life an occasion to reveal that the enigma of the end-of-life (of its point, purpose, or value) is our conscription to this deceit, to accept blindly and necessarily the lie that the meaning of life can be perpetuated forever.

This begins to point to the mix of pleasure and pain that Bataille observes in relating to oneself as both intimate and a thing, a mix driven by the necessity of self-objectification as "equipment for living." Now we might reformulate the wear and tear produced by modern society not as a simple attack upon the body by external forces but as a circuit needing to be placed in relation to Max Weber's (1930) comment on the "acquisition machine" of modern society driven to produce and acquire over and again as if living out Durkheim's (1951) anomic career of unending accumulation in the face of unfulfillable desire. If such a subject suffers the inner isolation Weber assumed, then we need to situate this relation in order to appreciate how the body can function as symptom or pretext in this circuit of solitude. This of course leads to a consideration of human anxiety (Blum 2011a, 222–29; Lacan 1981, 67–78; Miller 2006, 8–63; Ronen 2009, 77–106).

If we formulate anxiety on Lacanian lines as the sense of impotence in achieving separation as if one is forever and essentially condemned to the experience of indistinction and to the trace of formlessness that haunts any gesture of differentiation, we can imagine in this way how this apparent lack of consequentiality of any action makes inaction seem the only alternative. Thus, primary anxiety as a figure for the apprehension of what Nietzsche called the groundlessness of Being, could never be resolved by any relationship such as the family, love, or friendship because of the externality of all such relationships as chance encounters, as contingent, in ways that need to be supplemented and embraced by the absolutistic gesture that confers necessity upon them. This discloses the ever-present capacity for nihilism at the core of life, always capable of activation as part of a speculation imagining the point, purpose, and end-of-life. In the terminology of medicine, this capacity for nihilism is a chronic condition that, though never resolved, can be relieved through various symptoms. When Walter Benjamin (1969) says that death is the implicit topic of any story what he means is that any story of a life can be read as a tale testifying to the conquest of nihilism, and so, as a putting to rest of the temptation to fixate upon inaction and desolation. What this means in turn is that the social actor is engaged throughout life by the project of making over nihilism and the symptoms and secondary adjustments that this problem-solving makes necessary.

That is, if in certain respects end-of-life releases us from the hold of preoccupations, it also relieves us of commitment and of a tie to life since our rule by preoccupations is central and often obsessive. Then the freedom offered is also an occasion for anxiety as if the abundance of time, long sought and idealized as an objective, could be an occasion for painful reflection that was blocked or held in abeyance by the force and pleasure of preoccupation. If preoccupations are no longer sources of pleasure, the pleasure invested in Oedipal dreams of ambition and acquisition, the consequentiality of any present and future expectations, must be rethought in order to redistribute jouissance in different ways, making living in-itself, life without illusion, of consequence in the present. Improvisation taking shape as such redistribution must come to make meaning in a present. For example, the tie to worldly preoccupations, so patently meaningful as the game of life, is grounded in the Oedipal model of gain and loss, acquisition and competition, summarized in a logic of desire organized around a sense of life as a game to be won or lost. If what risks being recognized at end-of-life is that self-knowledge is of no consequence for winning or losing, the subject invariably faces the problem of making the desire for self-knowledge necessary and desirable in the face of its contingency. In terms of the life of the dying body, a subject needs to ask how to make life pleasurable in the absence of the game, that is, without illusion and dreams of winning and losing. Self-formation is invested in re-educating oneself to commitment to a present.

We can begin to identify the disintegrative experience of Falling Apart as itself a social phenomenon, and to explore such a relationship, we might ask who is most protected by the preoccupations of life and therefore who has most to lose when those preoccupations are relaxed or made transparent? In suggesting that Falling Apart seems to "strike," if we might use a disease metaphor, when a loss of innocence produces what Bataille calls a sense of betrayal and tendencies to act out for the betrayal by directing aggression against targets assumed to be responsible, then this "loss" is seen as if it creates the tendency to act-out as a disease. For example, the sociological classic by Henry and Short (Henry and Short 1954) assumed aggression to be externalized or internalized in the forms of homicide or suicide as kinds of diseases and they used "big data" in support of this hypothesis. To playfully engage such speculations, we might suggest that aggression could be directed towards oneself for not being strong enough to survive the trauma of such abandonment in the case of suicide and that homicide could be focused on targets either randomly identified as causes or systematically chosen as scapegoats. This might begin to show the impact of Falling Apart for views of terrorism, serial killing, and various similar sorts of attacks without using simple frustration-aggression explanations because of the complexity of the intervening variable of suffering and the fundamental ambiguity of repression, all pointing to the simplicity of causal stimulus-response models. In one case the self is seen as not strong enough to maintain one in the face of the disappointment following the loss of innocence, while in the other case, others are seen as strong enough to inflict such pain (but then again, if life is traumatic, its betrayal occurs for everyone in ways that make the use of others as scapegoats gratuitous and misleading). Perhaps what is thought is that others are responsible for misleading us to believe in life as mattering and now the betrayal exposes the lie as theirs. Whatever the account, Falling Apart makes manifest the experience of the abandonment of meaning in life as what Durkheim would call a social fact and how the kinds of "solutions" members develop to deal with such a problem must reveal the phenomenon as more than one attributable to having a bad day, a bad life, a bad upbringing, poverty, or any list of social determinants as eo ipso adequate, but as a value-added effect implicated in a complex rather than complicated system.

Cinematic Representations

I first became interested in Falling Apart as a phenomenon in watching Michael Douglas' careful choice of films that seemed to reveal a pattern in which the self-composition and self-confidence of a male protagonist was dramatically undermined by either a critical event, or disclosed as developing imperceptibly over time. I considered this type of film almost as a genre, not simply as an example of stories of alienated men, but seeming to resemble the tragic motif of a reversal of fortune involving a character of (relatively) high repute. Typically the reversal was attributed to financial failure, loss of power, or of affection. Yet the genre was also noticeable dramatically in representations of aging that appeared to involve no reversal of fortune but inevitable decline. It seemed important also that Falling Apart was resisted as a tragic genre because of the opinion that the model of tragedy cannot apply to a modern world since "high repute" cannot be represented in modern democratic times when the figure of any-man or of the common actor assumes precedence. Yet, there is a radical reversal of fortune in such films, which identify disintegration that seems apparent regardless of whatever we decide to call it.

Here the films that come to mind are organized around popular character actors besides Douglas such as Clint Eastwood, Jack Nicholson, George Clooney, and Richard Benjamin among others, all not simply portraying male victimization by predatory females as in many of Douglas' films, but as disruptions created by crises in work and domestic life. We want to rehabilitate Falling Apart as something other than a midlife crisis or seven year itch.

This relationship we represent as Falling Apart can be seen as linked to gender or conventionally, to what is called sex roles in terms of power, affection, and variables conventionally treated in sociology as indispensable in ways that dramatize their "loss" or diminution in power as traumatic and where the conception of whatever condition assumed to diminish the value of life is made sufficiently problematic as something to be possessed or lost as to put the problem of the point of life into question. In this way Falling Apart is typically represented as connected to an Oedipal imaginary relation to acquisition, possession and fear of loss, to anomie and castration, that invariably identifies its subject as acting out in compensatory ways for fear of dispossession or appetite for acquisition. In the way Durkheim asked of the subject of suicide how marriage protects men and women differently from this prospect, we could ask how men and women are defended differently from Falling Apart?

Thus, the genre can lead us to reflect on the representation of women seen as Falling Apart, recalling especially Herk Harvey's *Carnival of Souls*, *A Streetcar Named Desire*, Gena Rowland's character in *A Woman under the Influence*, and *Waltz With Me*. It seems that men and women in these cases are represented as Falling Apart differently in film, say in the contrast between the reversal of power of men, and the steady accretion of boredom and withdrawal in women, but when we focus upon literature, especially the novel, these differences start to be reconfigured. One proposition we might consider could address these differences between media, suggesting that ennui and boredom accentuated by a sensitivity to mortality begins to be discerned in male characters in novels as a trope decisively connected to aging. In terms of differences between media and gender, we might ask how male and female Falling Apart is represented for the reader in the novel, and for the spectator in the film. Would we expect a greater complexity in the portrayal of Falling Apart for the male character of the novel than in the film (a greater difference by media for men) than for the female character of the novel? The proposition that differences between male and female in representations of disintegration is greater in one medium compared to another is ungrounded and based on intuition but is certainly a line of inquiry following from these considerations.[1]

The problem of Falling Apart has been implicitly identified as the task a subject asks of and sets for oneself of how to make present now a past that seems lost, and how to make present now a future from which they will be separate? This is a version of Franz Rosenzweig's question that asked how can one live through a present while rejecting linear time? Here we expand Max Weber's notion of inner isolation to embrace not simply the lack of sociability in any present that is exemplified by his actor/subject of capitalism, but one's sense of being absent from the past and most important, from an unimaginable future.

Boredom

Benjamin was exercised by boredom and treated its experience as both the sign of an acute crisis, say as an historical moment, and as a chronic condition (that is intrinsic to the potentiality of a life in the sense that it is an apprehension, negative as it seems, that is always possible.) Benjamin even calls boredom a "malady" in ways that begin to connect it to the medical interest in the contrast between acute and chronic diseases.

> Boredom began to be experienced in epic proportions in the 1840s … typical illness of the time-weariness with life, deep depression, boredom.
>
> (Benjamin 1999, 111)

Benjamin reiterates the crisis as acute in relation to the ennui of romanticism, but references to Baudelaire and Nietzsche suggest that the experience coexists as part of the human condition (for Nietzsche in the recognition of the inexorable circularity of desire; for Baudelaire in the repetitiousness of the eternal in the temporal). Benjamin connects boredom to waiting: "Waiting is in a sense, the lined interior of boredom" (118). In identifying Baudelaire's antidote as the crowd, that "supreme remedy for boredom" (111, 115, 118) he creates the contrast between waiting and its distraction through exposure to enthusiasm as a paradigm for end-of-life as a battleground between privatization (waiting) and the public (crowd). Note how we are inquiring into the place of waiting and boredom in the embodied practices of the lived experience of aging and specifically how maturity seeks to be improvisational in relation to repetition. Consider further that if the means for realizing such an objective seems to be positive thinking, this is an interlocutor to the conception of maturity we are developing, simply an extreme opposite to resignation that we conceive improvisation to need to mediate. Thus, maturity has to "handle" the problem of repetitiousness (and the waiting and boredom it might elicit as responses) by negotiating the border between negativism and positive thinking (simple pessimism and simple optimism) to develop an improvisational relationship.

Games of Chance as a Lived Experience

In this respect, it is no accident that Benjamin was exercised by the coexistence of boredom and games of chance, especially gambling. Games of chance seem to rescue humans from inexorable boredom and its quintessential mode of adjustment in waiting. In some way, Baudelaire's crowd exemplifies the lure of the game of chance, adventure, surprise, fortuitous contingencies, and its happenstance as an antidote to boredom. Here, the pharmakon assumes a different disguise. Could the game of chance not also stand for the excess of jouissance, of self-transcendence, even self-destructive thymos, the need to reach beyond the finite by lathering oneself in the very vulgarity that can only be comic? Thus in life, waiting does not simply await death as the formula suggests, but could anticipate entertainment, excitement, the adventure, as what is just around the corner (Blum, 2003, Chapter 9). This means that a solution to the problem of death might lie in the capacity to imagine the adventure of the difference that promises to make a difference. Throughout, I have tried to imagine an ideal speaker as one who struggles to resist or subvert such common expectations that are elicited by the exhaustion of use value due to physical deterioration or by the dependencies and marginalization that create propensities towards privatization, segregation, and passivity. These are all intended solutions to the temptation to "fall apart."

If the game of chance is the paradigm we can use to model the lived experience, it could capture the movement of life as the fortuitous and contingent fluctuation of events that take shape in the impersonal and chance trajectories of conditions and the correlative opinions, preferences, and adjustments made to such a process. Baudelaire's crowd could be a figure for the lived experience as contingency and the appeal of the condition as both positive and as negative. In this way, the relationship to the crowd always needs something more, a desire to mediate and engage its turbulence through the force of intellect. This suggests that fundamental to the lived experience is its character as a relationship between chance, conditions, and imagination, disclosing the elementary structure of the lived experience to be the imaginative construal of contingency, of the condition (any condition), revealing the opportunism of imagination insofar as it accepts the fortuitous challenge of the Real as both opportunity and incentive. Imagination as a practice is revealed as such in any analysis that we do in which we track down a problem at first concealed from view but intimated in traces and clues that we uncover. Serendipity has been used to describe thinking as such a game, courting the unanticipated and hoping to seduce its appearance as if a surprising encounter. This is how we might call thinking an adventure.

The crowd seems to make reference to life and its necessary commitment to the enthusiasm of the present as "palliative care" while waiting appears as the living death. This suggests that the crowd be best formulated through the image of its volatility as a relationship to the emotions. While we might hate needing the crowd for relief (we hate needing and wanting the volatility of life as relief from the living death), we do desire modes and methods of imagining in ways that give us a singular voice in relation to its turbulence. We recognize that the crowd might be more than escapist distraction when we appreciate the types and adjustments it brings to view in the various shapes of enthusiasm towards its present, as material for the wide-awake actor and so, as the kaleidoscope Benjamin mentions that can only display this present as if a montage of unformed postures always remaining to be collected. In Benjamin's sense the crowd can be understood as usage, the language into which the poet plunges to secure his "booty."

Method: Rebeginning as Impasse Analysis

I try to exemplify in this book how we begin by listening to the voice of death in collective life as it materializes in a variety of views and images of a kind of elementary relationship. Baudelaire's crowd can certainly stand for this collection of voices as the immediate coming-to-view of the collective speech. In this sense we cooperate with death by listening to its registers and more specifically by observing how it is oriented to as a collection of opinions. Becoming an observer to the society and language of one's own is as long noted, to work at "suspending" participation through a refashioning that aims to adopt a degree of abstraction towards one's own familiar context. Such performance is to become an observer in such a way that requires a degree of eroticism in order to make oneself over into an objective figure capable of listening rather than simply and mechanically reacting by acting out. I stress that a thread linking the disparate opinions about the relationship to death is an image of a situation in which a subject seeks, often anxiously, to engage, calculate and/or master what is taken to be unknown. Such a subject must necessarily run up against the limits of language as Wittgenstein says or Lacan's wall of language, and it is such a collision for any particular concept that produces the aporia and the sensitivity it releases.

My approach assumes a togetherness and apartness in my own relationship to language and life, since I am both and simultaneously part of the language in which I intervene while also needing to create a distance that enables me to grasp its work as an expression of the movement of life. On the one hand, death is a representation to be worked out in life as a relationship. Similar to any notion as what is called a concept or a signifier, death is not an absolute that exists autonomously in relation to life and usage but is part of the movement of life itself and its conventional interpretive infrastructure and orthodoxa. Moreover, the word (even the brute fact death) must be seen to express something not just lexical but a path into a reflection upon the meaning of our action that is posited as such in some way. If death seems to occur as a brute fact or alien condition autonomous and separate from life and language, we still cooperate with this condition to make it seem as it is; that is, we cooperate with the notion by investing it with its meaning that materializes as whatever we take it to be.

This movement of the narrative strives to formulate the problem implicit as ground of the collective speech by listening to the surfaces and resonances, to the phraseology and its "beyond" that still exists within its folds. Such a drive both descriptive and more, in contrast to a stenographic record of the collective speech that is associated typically with describing, works to overcome this temptation by refashioning the text and by listening in ways that make observation itself somewhat of a performance. Such description works-through rather than repeats the collective speech (Freud's *durcharbeiten*) by imagining the orientation of the speaker through a gesture of exaggeration that takes delight in creating and inhabiting the voice as if ruled by a dream of realizing an ideal. Where Plato described ordinary empirical description from the perspective of the Sophist as if one "observing the moods and inclinations of a beast" (Plato 1941, 200–201, 492–493), a caretaker in that sense, an alternative approach travesties such a conception of description through an exaggeration as if a pornographer, trying to revive and make explicit the configuration of influences oft noted as unconscious and to refashion from its structure of associations its dreamwork. (See Marder 2013, 206, 210 for the dream and Beaujour 1981, 27–59 for the parameters of pornography and utopia that he assigns to the "strong" version of description.)

A review of John Barth's novels by Stephen Burn (2008) focuses on his method in a way that illustrates the model of impasse analysis that I am employing to animate the narrative of this work.

> Just as the idea of development provides his subject so it shapes many of his fictions, in which change does not bring resolution, but a step in a narrative moving towards a crucial crossroads. In several stories Barth initially creates a sense of traditional narrative coherence, only to amplify its conclusion with multiple branching possibilities… . Rejecting resolution, the story ends with a colon. This sets a pattern for the volume. The … stories begin with a question, and the plots move toward uncertainty. This open-ended structure connects the stories' form to their political and social agenda. Barth makes it clear that the approach of an ending does not narrow the range of options as much as it multiplies them. If we are living … trapped in a decadent society, then Barth invites us to resist the idea that the end is predetermined. Instead, he suggests, there is the possibility of briefly arising above the systems that surround us by an effort of mind, to evaluate them from a different perspective. To demonstrate this, he reworks the plot templates handed down to us with their rigid pattern of exposition-development-conclusion, by introducing an author figure who presents different ways of reaching several endpoints.
>
> (Burn 2008, 20–1)

In saying that Barth's stories begin with a question and move to uncertainty, he reiterates our beginning with the representation of a relationship (to death) as it is registered in a medley of speeches and opinions. The ending, as he says, multiplies "the range of options," which he demonstrates by "introducing an author figure" or what Impasse Analysis calls an ideal speaker, who "reworks" the rigid pattern of "exposition-development-conclusion" inherited in the discourse by showing the possibility of "rising above the systems" that seem to surround and constrain us in this interpretive infrastructure by orienting to them "from a different point of view." In a related way, my work is intended to develop from the statement of the impasse of the enigmatic relation of life to death as an original question not towards an interpretation that will bring our perplexity to an end, but in a way to a "rebeginning," in Barth's words, as a "chorus of voices (that) outline different paths the development might take," to a dream that might or might not live, introducing a "so what" refrain that seems to affirm the meaninglessness of human existence while "torn between the brevity and triviality of a human life, and the optimism of unfolding potential."

Conclusion

Hesiod permits us to begin to identify the elementary force of poetry as an aesthetic relation to writing.

> Fortunate is the man whom the muses love: sweet words flow from his lips. If someone has sorrow and is sick at heart and stunned with fresh trouble on his mind, and if a servant of the Muses sings of the glorious deeds of men in former times or of the blessed gods whose home is Olympus, he quickly forgets his bad thoughts and no longer remembers his troubles: the gift of these goddesses instantly divert the mind.
>
> (56, ii, 116–153)

Here, poetry is said to originate as an eventful collision with the unruly emotions (the crowd) as an attempt at amelioration not by denying or reducing the emotions but through the pleasure offered by "sweet words" in ways that might divert the mind. This primordial vision of art portrays the shepherd, the one isolated in the wilds, as surrounded by ghostly spirits in the "luminous night" (Nietzsche), who can be touched by the music of speech. In this elementary situation music and language come together as song, and with the aid of the muses, help make magic. We see that the magic is nothing other than what Jacques Rancière depicts as the aesthetic relationship to the world, the need and desire to commit to form as part of a disengagement from the tyranny of conditions that seem to determine us, to commit to the "absolute humour" (Baudelaire) that knows its limits even as it pursues a way of living dependent upon the imaginary of unlimitedness *hic et nunc*. Whatever the relation to death, whether it serves as a good or bad object, the tumult of the emotions remains to be addressed, explored, and healed as an unalterable condition that we are not free to disregard, the consequences of which we inherit as if a legacy of the object (death) itself much like its destiny. If death is linked irreparably to the volatility of the emotions, the visualization of such a relationship might just escape or exceed all attempts to make it visible and to confirm or test its reality only and exclusively through such means and methods. What is death must exceed any conditions enumerated to determine it as a corporeal fact with beginning and end, for death must exceed such conditions as an object of desire, an object neither "subjective" nor "objective" but an object of destiny (Baudrillard, 1987).

Certainly, theorizing death has to pay its respects to the experience disclosed as sorrow, being "sick at heart," and "stunned with fresh trouble in the mind." Taking our lead from Hesiod, we might be able to glimpse the prospect of a relationship to the object, to death in this case, not simply in its capacity to defend oneself from anxiety by escape or denial but through an engagement with language mediated by the desire to remake this eventful encounter with the music of "sweet words" in representing any and every relationship to being "sick at heart."

This is how Baudelaire can express contempt for those who are bored by the crowd and immune to its stimulation. This is because the crowd is our data in any present, the "matter" which we must develop and to which we need relate. The crowd as such usage is the rudimentary way in which the society speaks, creating in its common currency the opportunity for self-disclosure and mutually oriented social action (Weber, 1947). Thus, what the crowd brings to view in its volatility is nothing substantive such as the content of its objectives and hankerings, but the play of uncollectedness and dispersion itself that might always be engrossing as an opportunity for one to recover voice in such a medley, to maintain a space for sovereignty by endeavoring to find oneself in such dispersion, engaging the resistance offered by such a mix by testing oneself as a player in its game of chance. The crowd brings to view the lower order ruling any present, the ludicrous spectacle of finitude at this historical moment in the context of any present, the inertia that treats its repetition as an advance. What is absolutely comic is that one's sense of superiority to the crowd is cancelled by recognition of a fundamental unity and togetherness, that the knowledge that sets one apart is cancelled by the ignorance that brings us together, that our appearance of inequality is the work of fortuna. This means that reflective practice itself (such as theorizing) could and should be oriented to as a game of chance that imitates the contingent and fortuitous workings of the Real and that this could be highlighted at the end-of-life when the ambiguity of the Real comes to view. What the game reveals is that despite any differences between winners and losers, the rules are set by the machine of Oedipus (loss, gain, acquisition). If maturity grasps this verity, it might be a way of formulating the objective for care as an embodiment of maturity, for example, a capacity to reflect upon dementia as an attempt to solve this problem. In this respect, I conclude this chapter with the story of another writer who can prepare us to care for speech that we are tempted to find unintelligible.

> One day I'll be out walking with my brother in the place in my being where I once had my poet friend by my side … where I'm thinking very hard about

The Squirrel ... I'll want to tell him the beginning. One fine morning in October 1964, death was starting up again, one is out walking alive, out of the blue, death turns up. Washington Square cemetery, "submission to the inner reality" my friend said, he was smiling at the idea of the end, I staggered, seeing the cadaver of a squirrel half-buried in the ground, as if it had hurried to hide its death in Hell but, taken by surprise as it was going down, it remained stuck there like an inhabitant of Herculaneum "this is the secret of art" my friend the American poet said, I staggered, seeing in the cadaver's half-body the annunciation of the fate of my poet friend. I saw two dead. I know, I fear it in vain, ever since Washington Square, I live on the dead. "Submission to the door of the book" says my friend. "Pass death and there's literature. Descend underground, follow the squirrel, it will take you to the root of the secrets." So there are gods with short lives, I tell myself, for Homer the gods come into our beds with the grace of the young things in novels, in Manhattan Hector is a squirrel, or maybe it was Fabrice. In those days I'll tell my brother, I worshipped the friend and the squirrel with the same terror. I saw life I saw death. I saw life: I saw death. That's all I have to say.

(Cixous (2008) 2011, 31–32)

Note

1 Films of Fassbinder, novels by Jean Rhys, and Calvino's Mr. Palomar are very good examples of this discourse that I have explored in classes.

References

Bataille, Georges. (1973) 1989. *Theory of Religion.* Translated by Robert Hurley. New York: Zone Books.

Baudelaire, Charles. 1972. "The Painter of Modern Life." In *Selected Writings on Art and Artists*, translated by P.E. Charvet, 390–436. Cambridge: Cambridge University Press.

Benjamin, Walter. (1936) 1969. "The Work of Art in the Age of Mechanical Reproduction." In *Illuminations: Essays and Reflection,* edited by Hannah Arendt, translated by Harry Zohn. New York: Schocken Books, 217–252.

——. 1999. *The Arcades Project.* Edited by Rolf Tiedemann. Translated by Howard Eiland and Kevin McLaughlin. Cambridge, MA: Belknap Press of Harvard University Press.

Blum, Alan. 2003. *The Imaginative Structure of the City*. Montreal: McGill-Queen's University Press.

——. 2008. "Preserving the Notion of Preservations: The Ineradicable Perpetuity of Me, Myself and I." In *The Venice Charter Revisited: Modernism, Conservation and Tradition in the 21st Century,* edited by Matthew Hardy, 125–138. Cambridge: Cambridge Scholars Publishing.

——. 2011a. *The Grey Zone of Health and Illness*. Bristol: Intellect Press.

——. 2011b. "Life, Death and the In-Between: The Duck/Rabbit and the Face of the Clown." In *Spectacular Death: Interdisciplinary Perspectives on Mortality and (Un) representability*, edited by Tristanne Connolly, 21–41. Bristol: Intellect Press.

——. 2013. "Age as a Social Form: The Phenomenology of the Passage." *Journal of Medical Humanities* 35 (1): 19–36.

——. 2014. "The Ordeal of Solitude." *History of the Human Sciences* 27 (2): 118–132.

——. 2015. "The Border Between Intimacy and Anonymity in Innocuous Action: The Greeting as a Social Form." *Journal of Classical Sociology* 16 (1): 69–83.

Burke, Kenneth. 1957. *The Philosophy of Literary Form: Studies in Symbolic Action.* Berkeley, CA: University of California Press.

Burn, Stephen. 2008. "'Much adieu': Review of J. Barth, The Development." Pg. 20 in *Times Literary Supplement*, October 17 2008.

Cixous, Hélène. (2008) 2011. *Hemlock: Old Women in Bloom.* Translated by Beverley Bie Brahic. Malden, MA: Polity Press.

Dumm, Thomas. 2008. *Loneliness as a Way of Life*. Cambridge, MA: Harvard University Press.

Durkhiem, Emile. 1951. *Suicide: A Study in Sociology.* Edited by George Simpson. Translated by John A. Spaulding and George Simpson. New York: Glencoe.

Freud, Sigmund. (1917) 1957. "Mourning and Melancholia." In *Volume 11, On Metapsychology: The Theory of Psychoanalysis*, translated by James Strachey, 245–268. London: Penguin.

Henry, Andrew and James Short. 1954. *Suicide and Homicide*. Glencoe, Ill: Free Press.

Lacan, Jacques. 1981. "The Split Between the Eye and the Gaze," in *The Seminar of Jacques Lacan Book XI: The Four Fundamental Concepts of Pyschoanalysis*, 67–78. Edited by Jacques-Alain Miller, translated by Alan Sheridan. New York: W.W. Norton and Co.

——. 2006. "The Subversion of the Subject and the Dialectic of Desire in the Freudian Unconscious," in *Ecrits*, 671–702. Translated by Bruce Fink. New York: W.W. Norton and Co.

Marder, Elissa. 2013. "Real Dreams." *The Southern Journal of Philosophy* 51, Spindel Supplement: 196–213.

Miller, J.A. 2006. "Introduction to reading Jacques Lacan's Seminar on Anxiety II." *lacanian ink* 27: 8–63.

Ronen, Ruth. 2009. *The Aesthetics of Anxiety*. New York: State University of New York Press.

Simmel, Georg. 1950. "Knowledge, Truth, and Falsehood in Human Relations" in *The Sociology of Kurt Wolf*, edited and translated by Kurt H. Wolff, 307–316. New York: The Free Press.

——. 1955. *Conflict and the Web of Group Affiliations.* Translated by Kurt H. Wolff and Reinhard Bendix. Glencoe, IL: The Free Press.

Weber, Max. (1905) 1930. *The Protestant Ethic and the Spirit of Capitalism.* Translated by Talcott Parsons. London: George Allen & Unwin.

Part II

Dementia and the Look of Madness—Aging, Raging, and the Poetics of Passing On

In this section I use the tension in care elicited by the need to relate to the intimate suffering aroused by so-called dementia as an occasion to examine how neurological fantasies compelled by biomedicine work very specifically to reroute anxieties over death, conceivable both for the sufferer and for the one who cares for this vulnerable subject. I suggest that dementia can be understood not simply as the progressive deterioration of the body and its neurological disintegration but as the process through which a human subject is infected by an awareness of mortality and the images of inevitable limitation and loss that it summons to mind. Far from being a sign of corporeal weakness, the symptoms revealed in dementia can point to a degree of enlightened helplessness for one trying to solve the impossible problem of existence in time between a past that is lost and a future that must appear inscrutable.

When caregiving takes its bearings from a neurological framework it tends to foreclose attentiveness to the subjectivity of the suffering, disguising its own inarticulateness and anxiety over mortality in digestible and reassuring formats. Care for the lived experience of the dying body requires something other than palliatives of positive thinking or medical science, but a curriculum that can orient to the experience of a self attuned to the inevitable loss of life, care trying in its way to cultivate a shared jouissance of suffering between witness and intimate. I pose the question of how or whether care is possible under such conditions and if it is possible to mobilize affect in both witness and other for an innovative relationship to desperation. I claim mortality and its complexity as the unspoken and taboo topic of this situation, using the case of dementia to explore what Baudrillard calls the molecular idealism of materialist doctrine, and the ways it affects caregivers from rationalization to depression. As an antidote, I suggest the novel as an important resource for representing the lived experience of dying for those who care and feel separated, as a resource for a curriculum of witnessing.

7 The Enigma of the Brain and its Place as Cause, Character, and Pretext in the Imaginary of Dementia

Introduction

An analysis of the collective engagement with the disease known as Alzheimer's and the dementia reputed of it reveals recourse to a socially standardized formula that attributes causal agency to the brain in the absence of clinching knowledge. I propose that what Baudrillard calls the model of Molecular Idealism stipulates such a neurological view of determinism in order to provide caregivers with reassurance in the face of the perplexing character of dementia and the depressing reactions to mortality that it brings to the surface.

Biomedical Anxiety

The biomedical formulation of dementia as a brain or cognitive disturbance permits all concerned to avoid rethinking the bizarre behavior of the subject in relation to the depressing experience of mortality and of dying as the inevitability it is, and so, of considering the affected person as depressed rather than as undergoing a period of somatic deterioration. This unspoken assumption of biomedical research, its assignment of causal priority to the body, permits all involved to avoid reflecting upon death as what we might call the "real" object of concern. Thus, the research "acts out" a primary fear of death and its overtones, possibly misrecognizing depression as the corporeal deterioration that is as likely to be a symptom as a cause. What becomes contagious in ways that can afflict caregivers, as well as those for whom they care, is the unfathomable character of death and of its inevitability as a condition to endure.

In this chapter, I use end-of-life as a case to investigate how aging under modern conditions is identified as a regime or order that structures expectations around the "fact" of an unthought relationship between advancing years and physical deterioration that tends to imagine the category as homogeneous despite individual variations that, when conceded, are assumed to be unified by the problems that senility sets. For example, from the perspective of medical care and most conceptions of caregiving, what the uniqueness of the person contributes to the condition (of agedness) needs to be disregarded or held in abeyance as particular, in order to conduct efficient care. The easiest way to enforce standardized conceptions upon a diverse population is to imagine them as collectible by neurological or genetic factors that then work to free the investigator from having to confront the conundrum of meaning that is invariably dramatized in any engagement with an individual. The body then seems to function as a way of relieving anxiety over the question of meaning. For example, the notion of sickness as a role, of the sick role, associates illness with the motivation of the subject and practitioner, always eliciting concerns over the secondary gain of illness for the patient, asking after reasons for cooperation and "non-adherence" in ways that point to the complexity of the relation and how this compromises simple causal accounts. For sociology, at least, much more is involved in collective relationships and representations of health and illness than inventories of somatic causes and the intellectual relief and relaxation that such research seemed to produce.

In the history of the human sciences the mind-body problem has appeared in different guises in ways that affect all theorizing on social action and with respect to stages in the life cycle. Such theorizing materializes in models of conduct and claims to knowledge, in the identification of norms, rules, and policies to guide distinguishing, and in conceptions of the subject and of typical experiences of an order (see Blum 2011, 149–166).

In this sense, the imaginary of the brain as an agent in behavior has been used in all sorts of ways, even outside medicine, to compensate for a failure of analytic capacity to grasp the apparently unfathomable experience presented by a subject. Just as artists regularly rhapsodize over the brain as an elegant and complex bit of machinery, sophisticated philosophers appeal to it when confronting the enigma of the future or of an afterlife in contemplating death, and others enthuse over the promise of neurological research in unraveling the mysteries of addiction or the phenomenology of any action.

The Brain as a Character in the Discourse on End-of-Life

The use of the brain in explanatory formulae collects a variety of interests around the functions of disavowing responsibility and limiting the agency of all parties. The impersonality of the brain alleviates fear for the behavior being seen as "personal" or "subjective," and the complications that seem to offer objections that have to be accounted for within the context of a plurality of different possibilities. As Wittgenstein ([1953] 1958) would say, asserting "the brain did it!" seems to resolve the ambiguity for all concerned. The brain then serves as a locus of collectivization that can bring together in its topos a range of interests, pacifying the frustration and tension likely to arise between interpreters over the meaning of a phenomenon and its representation as a force in life.

I propose then that it is inefficient to listen to the patient without factoring in subjectivity because this simplifies any exchange when subjectivity is banned or foreclosed. In terms of caregiving in dementia, the recipe is passed on to the caregivers of the "demented" as a set of rules of thumb for guiding them in relating to the enigma of intersubjectivity. These formulae speculate after-the-fact about brain dysfunctions, based upon post-mortem observations of the brain, making inferences about causality from the presence of noted irregularities. Yet there can be no demonstration that the irregularity "caused" the bizarre behavior since there can be no controlled observation of onset. In such a climate it is reasonable to expect all concerned to show symptoms of depression, and especially caregivers who might only be impotent in the face of such startling reversals in the behavior of intimates.

The Brain as Object of Desire: Popular Enthusiasm

The collective fascination with thought, institutionalized in part in the disciplines and conventions of philosophy and psychology, has typically risked abstraction on the one hand and banality on the other. Throughout, the dark side of thought, seeming irrational, inaccessible, or an excess beyond the imaginary capacities of humans to objectify, could only come to view in actions appearing disorderly, distorted in various shapes, whether as evil, eccentricity, criminality, or madness. Yet in no way was the figure of the brain celebrated as it is today in any and all accounts of conduct. Thus, if the Greek epic includes tales of heroism, and the tragedies of self-destructive actions, commentators rarely confronted such action neurologically. The actions of madness, even of butchers and assassins and of culprits such as those judged at Nuremberg, or great tyrants and dictators, rarely had a neurological eye cast upon them (except for the occasional eccentric work that offered to plunge in where angels feared to tread). Indeed, even the Not-Guilty-by-Reason-of-Insanity verdict rarely seemed to employ such a model.

In this respect, we might ask why now the brain comes to be factored into accounts of dementia when the actions of persons appear bizarre and incoherent and when there is no really compelling evidence for its causal status, nothing except publicity over its research "advances" that remain descriptive and of limited inferential value. I want to pose the problem of the uses of the brain as a trope in such accounts and its possible function as a paradigm for those who easily employ it as second nature, as part of their habituated reactions to what is perplexing and enigmatic in human conduct. For example, in taking up the problem of caregiver responses to age-related dementia, it seemed as if the depression and frustration constantly reported by the caregivers (whether family or semi-professionals) was connected to what appeared to be the enigmatic and irrational behavior of the suffering subjects, registered in a disorderliness that made it difficult for caregivers to find their footing. What was noted recurrently was an unthought allegiance among all concerned to a modal explanation of the hallucination, positing it to be the result of neurological dysfunctions, and particularly the brain. While neurology and medical science would attribute this resurgent focus upon the brain to advances in medical science and neurological research, this presupposes what we are inquiring into, especially if we are reserved towards these accomplishments as anything more than limited inferences based upon post-mortem findings and data.

I propose to examine concerns for the care of age-related dementia as a public health issue and a problem for caregivers as part of a discourse on the so-called breakdown of thought as reflected in an apparent incoherence that interpreters seem helpless to engage and endure, requiring under such conditions new and more palpable information.

Given the furor over the enigma of dementia in Alzheimer's disease (Kolata 2010), and especially the concern for depression among caregivers, for example (see Galvin *et al.* 2010; Bielski 2010), we can ask how the use of the body in both research and lay accounts factors into the collective representation and fascination as something other than a "hard fact" but as a possible sign of the different intuitions of mortality that separate caregiver from demented and from the need to find reassurance through genetic and somatic speculation. If the condition is reputed to arouse fear over "the erosion of selfhood" (Kontos 2006, 195), it can also be expected to inspire a search for socially organized ways of living with such an anxiety, what Kenneth Burke (1957) called "equipment for living." Thus, Kontos notes "Alzheimer's disease is regarded as the most bewildering and frightening condition facing the aging population in the twenty-first century" (Schroeder *et al.* 1990, quoted in Kontos 2006, 195), that it is "described as a living death … a private hell of devastation" (195). Such a fear then can be assumed to create not only medical problem-solving, but socially oriented ways of handling the fear itself. This suggests that the research directed to solve the problem of Alzheimer's cannot stand apart as if a neutral technology administered by a medically attuned expertise but becomes part of the social organization of such equipment for living. In this chapter, I will begin to lay out ways of conceiving of care as a discourse in order to make some of these problems transparent.

The Medical Imaginary and the Dream of Research

> Researchers are finding simple and accurate ways to detect Alzheimer's long before there are definite symptoms. In addition to spinal fluid tests they also have new PET scans of the brain that show the telltale amyloid plaques that are a unique feature of the disease. And they are testing hundreds of new drugs that, they hope, might change the course of the relentless brain cell death that robs people of their memories and abilities to think and reason.
>
> (Kolata 2010, paragraph 5)

Here, researchers are encouraged to test the population to determine in advance if they have signs of the disease in the absence of any knowledge (before the fact) of what is unique to the disease.

But these "telltale amyloid plaques" can only be discovered in ways that render their causal status problematic, even if detected in living subjects, and that seriously compromise the boast that such conditions are "a unique feature of the disease." The desire to collect sufferers as if they constitute a unified category is demanded by the need for standardized approaches and treatment that itself is required by the logistics of processing quantities of people. The very category of Alzheimer's disease is designed to collect all, without respect for variations introduced by the singularity of persons collected, and it can only be produced as such by basing the category upon an externalized condition such as brain dysfunction. If individual variations are noted after the fact, then they can best be attributed to other biological, chemical, or neurological factors ad infinitum. The mind and "mental" can only be regarded as a foreign intruder that interrupts the objective of molecular idealism to begin with a population purified through standardization of any extraneous conditions of "subjectivity." Collecting, instructed by the need to find properties shared by disparate individuals, locates such properties after the fact in an imaginary conception of the brain and the distribution of its salient features. Thus, it is the desire to discover "unique features" that produces these features as unique and telltale in perfect accord with Baudrillard's notion of simulation that the sociologist W. I. Thomas (1928, 572) long ago called the Self-fulfilling Prophecy: "If we define a situation as Real, then it is Real in its consequences."

The desire to discover a unique feature in the brain posits as Real whatever feature in the brain they decide to identify as unique. Medical science, driven by the desire to find a unique feature in the brain, *will* find a feature in the brain and call it unique. As in Baudrillard's ([1977 and 1981] 1983) discussion, it is the model that determines the discovery by affirming itself as Real.

> Only affiliation to the model makes sense and nothing flows any longer according to its end, but precedes from the model, the "signifier of reference," which is a kind of interior finality and the only resemblance there is.
>
> (101)

> Such is the "mystic elegance of the binary system, of the zero and the one," from which all being precedes. Such is the status of the sign that is also the end of signification.
>
> (106)

> Finality no longer belongs to the term; there is no longer a term, nor a determination. Finality is there beforehand inscribed in the code.
>
> (108–109)

> [T]hat delirious illusion of uniting the world under the aegis of a single principle… . The fascination of the biological, of the biomedical, dates from the very beginnings of science.
>
> (110)

> [S]cience has selected itself as generating formula, a model discourse, upon the faith of a conventional order (not just any, however; that of total reduction).
>
> (114)

It is not the conventionality of this cybernetic definition of life that Baudrillard contests, but the way the subject of medical science is tempted to treat a formula as absolute, making the imaginary of such "molecular idealism" a necessity rather than a convention whose terms, conditions, and signification need to be engaged. The either/or model bans the complexity of the signifier, its determination, and finality, as external to the code. This automated piety towards the code denies the very antipathy to superstition and ideology that science has long affirmed. We see this dramatically in the astonishing accounts of dementia in Alzheimer's disease as if the closing of the books on the priority of the brain leaves space only for technical refinements, or self-help manuals for explaining the situation to caregivers.

Baudrillard's conception of the model conceives of it as a symbolic order or method that creates and establishes a social world and its jurisdiction. This is a standard and long-time resource of the sociology of knowledge that treats the normative order represented as the rules of social action in some domain as a social world in microcosm, populated by actors, courses of action, environmental relevances and the like in necessary accord with the unspoken emphases of the system and its priorities. This itself is no news, long a staple of phenomenology, the work of Alfred Schutz ([1953] 1973), Harold Garfinkel's ethnomethodology (1967), and many influences. What is stressed is the function of the model as a method for seeing and selecting, and so, as a tool for managing affairs. Baudrillard's specific genius lay in noting the character of any social arrangement as such a model and method, for example the amusement park set up as Disneyland. Enabled to see Disneyland not simply as an innocent facility, but as a manner and method of organizing the world, he would go the further step of appreciating its rules or regulations as a code that structures expectations and orientations among and between those affected by it, as a microcosm instructing desire and notions of desirability, success, failure, and the distribution of enumerable e/affects. For our purposes, what is important is Baudrillard's claim that the finality of the production of the model is dissolved in (what he calls) the series, in other words, that the origin and ground of the model is disregarded and superseded by concerns for its standardization, making the message of the model its method, lying in its use and dissemination, in its reproduction. This is a perfect translation of McLuhan's (1964) mantra, the medium is the message, that all media are methods for structuring expectations.

Molecular Idealism

The model starts from an assumption that dementia is a loss of mind, and instead of approaching this as an interrogative terrain, assumes immediately that whatever is seen as lost is produced by the brain, by aging, or by deterioration. In the absence of an engagement with the meaning of the situation, the prayer of molecular idealism is repeated. What mind is assumed to lose is its mastery over the body by virtue of changes that are seen as interrupting the normal expectation of such mastery. Mind is expected to use the body rationally by adjusting to its demands through habituation as if the mind rationally adapts to exigencies introduced by the body and to the changes it presents, whether in normal development, sudden disease, or cases such as aging, where change (such as decline) is expected to be adapted to and normalized. Accordingly, this view of the loss of mind treats the loss as determined by the body in ways that cause mind to send a message to the body to take over control. In contrast to Freud ([1895] 1957), the relation of mind to body and back again is treated typically as text messaging in ways that foreclose any sense of an intersubjective relation, a model that complies with a notion of the body as the command control center of the mind. Playing off the model of the revolution in which the old regime attempts to influence the body to assume power because of mind's failure to govern itself, this view could also be seen as a result of the mind's use of body for self-defense by enlisting the support of the body through its displaced habituation in the symptom. This is not only a model of re-presentation based upon an image of a mercenary relationship, but of a means-end alliance and delegation of authority in accordance with a variety of canonical tropes on political representation (see Blum 2011, 191–211).

It should be noted that the celebration of the brain is not at all based upon clinching empirical evidence, or even on post-mortem inferences as mentioned, but, at best, upon results of "high-resonance imaging" (Quenqua 2011, paragraph 10) that show physical changes in the brain to be co-present with some symptom (e.g. addiction) in a way that testifies to the researcher that the condition can be managed "much like the management of other chronic diseases" (Alford quoted in Quenqua 2011, paragraph 11), transforming the notion of "chronicity" to the body rather than to the mind. Note the interpretive strings being pulled here: managing the disease through drugs (due to noticing a pattern, the relation of the symptom to such effects) is taken as grounds for a neurological view that could as well apply to many activities where change might be noted after the symptom, for example, eating, divorce, swimming, bankruptcy, concert-going, road-rage, being in love, writer's block, losing a job. Molecular idealism would treat such effects as "stress" instead of orienting to the effects as occasions to rethink the place of the symptom in a life, by rethinking the particularity of such affect in this shape for this life (using the "brain" in an account of writer's block just as in alcoholism enables the sufferer to disavow any examination of this relationship in which he/she is implicated because it is deemed most important to eliminate the symptom rather than engage it thoughtfully). If MRI imaging reveals changes in the brain after such activities, this does not warrant the conclusion that the brain is a causal factor in the onset of such activities, though it might suggest that such activities could be managed through medication. The idea that behavior might be changed through drugs is meant to celebrate the impotence of self-reflection as a mechanism of behavioral change, assuming the addict or depressive wants relief from the symptom at any cost even without understanding what attracts him/her to the behavior in the first place. Molecular idealism treats itself as "succeeding" with respect to self-reflection because it is more efficient at managing the course and withdrawal of symptoms. Thus, the battleground here is over the best relationship to the symptom and whether a discursive relationship has any value compared to the technological methods of symptom extinction and manipulation that have been imagined as most effective over the years and coveted in every totalitarian regime (the hidden persuaders always seen as functioning behind the scenes as sensory operators). I am not suggesting that molecular idealism has an "ideological" purpose as latent compared to its manifest activities, but rather that the formula in practice lays the ground and lends its support to the celebration of an inverse relation between reflective thought and change. From this angle, the intuition of mortality and its inevitability to which the aged are bound to be drawn can also be treated as a disturbing symptom, a disease to be managed, instead of an occasion for reflection. If we think of death as in need of pain relief and efficient management through pharmaceutical measures, many would agree to this for everyone hates being in the presence of such melancholy. In a certain way, molecular idealism can then proceed to relieve the world of all negative thinking, provided it is discomforting to those who "suffer" in such ways and that all might agree that it is better to purge the symptom than risk its unstable and irregular reappearance.

Custody as Customer Care and Witnessing as Attunement

The risk of stereotyping the aged was dramatized in the case of the dementia sufferer by the unreflective acceptance of somatic causes, because research shows caregivers to be perplexed and frustrated by the bizarre behavior. In this sense, formulaic views of dementia, both in research and formats for caregivers, lead me to question how the attribution of the enigmatic disease to somatic or genetic causes might be a way of assuaging the anxiety of caregivers, a secondary gain that could avoid thinking about the distress of the sufferer who begins to glimpse the inevitability of death.

This begins to dramatize the difference between two relations to bad conditions (whether dementia, disease, or the crisis of aging), between what we can think of as a custodial relation and bearing witness. The expectation here is that the use of the body and its dysfunctions as a formula in such accounts serves to relieve the anxiety of the caregiver by providing a degree of certainty in a situation where such attribution can exempt one from personal responsibility for having to engage the complex question of the meaning of the hallucination for everyone, allowing the caregiver to become in this respect a custodian charged with maintaining the encounter, rather than one engaged by the need to translate the formula and to try to grasp its implications for the kind of life they have had together.

Implications of Different Models of Mind and Body Relations

Here are two ways of thinking of the rule of mind over body. In the first case, mind rules body insofar as body always needs to be represented as such, even in its guise as the most incorrigible and indubitable condition. The fact that the mind is and was always lost is the model of the unconscious, meaning that anything happening in the way of the body as a condition or interruption of the course of a life, even as an incorrigible and indisputable intervention, still needs to be represented, i.e. perceived and integrated, in ways that feed back and become part of the self-understanding of the person. That is, if the childhood disease and its obvious somatic base seems the best example of a separable, external effect or invasion, its connection to the person, the necessity of connecting its exteriority to its intimacy as an oriented object for all engaged, expresses the place of seeing-as, in ways always problematic as ongoing interpretive work. As we have already suggested, in the second case, mind uses body to defend itself against conditions (not just in post-traumatic responses, but in the work of converting any significant anxiety-producing condition). This is Freud's ([1895] 1957) hysteria model.

We appreciate the work and interaction of such notions in discussions of aging that typically treat the response of mind to the deterioration forced by body as the limitation of volition by determinism, and the attempt of impotence to redeem what is lost through fantastic images (such as the hallucinations and scrambled thought of dementia). One of the forceful images connecting to aging as a decline of capacities is the conception of the subject as either determined in a mechanical way, or as conditioned to the point of desiring to recover what was lost (to resurrect vestiges of potency in substitute objects, or reveries of restoring mastery). Most typically, aging is viewed as a holding-on operation in which nothing more than maintenance is desired.

It is essential to recognize how the very "fact" of decline is represented as such in the self-representation of the aged in ways that seem to appropriate and so confirm the medical model of somatic deterioration. The aged, always seeming to execute the script, tend to do what is expected of them (or in some cases, seeming eccentric, transgress). Thus, the aged represent themselves in the formulaic ways suggested by the regime of the symbolic order, depicting the trajectory as a loss, with this self-representation becoming part of the subject and its desire to meet expectations and to live according to the law. This self-fulfilling prophecy can interact with the decline, accentuating it in descriptions of memory loss, incompetence, and indifference, as if these accounts are designed to meet the requirements of the formula. For example, instabilities in everyday life, such as misplacing keys, slips of the tongue, accidents at home and driving, are seen as infractions that are telling effects of somatic deterioration even as such effects are pervasive and omnipresent for all and sundry. Most important, the babble of speech unhinged is treated as a sign that reiterates the deterioration.

Losing One's Mind and the Euphemism of Stress

In the varied accounts of the loss of mind in age-related dementia, the causal preeminence of the brain does not require the disappearance of mind. In this model, mind becomes reconfigured as the self-relating orientation to such a priority, the capacity to endure and live with the damaged brain. Loss of mind then means the loss of any capacity for self-direction in this sense, or better, the loss of the illusion that mind has (what Freud calls) an executive function rather than servile status. As such an increasing awareness even under conditions of extreme deterioration, mind can be celebrated as a limited shape of agency in relation to the stress of bearing a damaged body. Mind is reconfigured as the capacity to knowingly inherit the burden of stress, and care is directed to this condition. Thus, if the medical student might major in medical education, the minor subject could be legitimated as cultivating an approach to the patient suffering the stress of the condition. Note that for Freud, mind did not have such a secondary or derivative status as a reaction to the body and the illness, because it was conceptualized as part of the dynamic of becoming ill through the figure of the symptom and its dialectic. Mind as the stress of living with dementia, of having to adapt to its "stress," is not akin to Freud's conception of the minded relation to anxiety that uses the body for converting the threat into habituated conduct.

This conception of mindfulness or limited agency is reflected in the movement to patient-centered care that seeks to correct the limits of biomedical reductionism (Brooker 2003; Cottrell and Schulz 1993; Kitwood 1997), seeking to remedy what is seen as depersonalization by more personal engagements with patients, trying to recover the person behind the patient, or the self masked in images of its disembodiment (Kitwood 1997; Kontos and Naglie 2007).

> We advocate a new care ethic that underscores the importance of the communicative capacity of the body to enrich our imagination and connect us to the personhood of others, thereby fostering sympathetic and person-centred dementia care.
>
> (Kontos and Naglie 2007, 551)

The cases they analyze are all examples of caregivers coming to recognize personal characteristics of sufferers, where selfhood seems to be expressed in enumerable ways through various preferences, forms of social etiquette, habits, obsessions, and the like (see Kontos and Naglie 2007, 550–561). These expressions of selfhood, whether verbal or nonverbal, are taken as self-evident signs of the person, as for example: "the way that persons with dementia unthinkingly carry and project their bodies with coherence; the often subtle attentiveness to their appearance, cleanliness, and social etiquette; bodily expressions of class distinction; and the spontaneity to their actions" (565). Here, the person is reputed to materialize beyond the mask of the category when we can view the body as information-bearing and as a display in this sense. Yet, as this convention has long acknowledged, such impression management can only be the beginning of analysis, always requiring formulative work that develops its character as more than testimonials for agency, but as action (in Weber's [1921–1922] 1947 sense) that is "oriented to an order and governed in its course."

So, in exactly the same way that the body can be said to function as a formula for ascribing dementia, we might suggest that this notion of person-centered care can risk functioning, even in its good-hearted attempt to awaken the sensitivity of caregiver to the person, as a format that forecloses further analysis. In other words, the emotional rapport mobilized by sensitivity for the person in these limited senses of respect for agency, or dignity, can actually limit the analytic capacities of caregivers. In contrast to the positive uses of emotional rapport for caregiving, I am rekindling the possible negative capabilities of the counter-transference in the relationship, by suggesting that we need to revisit the conception of the missing person in dementia as something deep rather than shallow (say, as something other than the need to recognize "personality"). In contrast to what is called patient-centered care, we might begin to think of a notion of witnessing that focuses on the analysis of resistances in the relationship, rather than on cultivating a pacific exchange of information and support.

The Lear Effect

In this respect, my research (2011) on death and aging proposed that the hallucinations of aging people suffering Alzheimer's or vascular dementia, typically attributed to genetic or somatic functions or to cognitive impairment (Iemolo *et al.* 2009; Galvin *et al.* 2010; Mittleman *et al.* 2004) can alternatively be engaged by reading/listening to the hallucination as an attempt to express the unfathomable experience of dying and the impossible imagining of death (Blum 2011) in ways destined to be incoherent to those paternal (medicine), or confused (caregivers), who can only treat it abstractly, or to those who want to compensate with kindness for the bureaucratization of care. The proposition was discovered by talking to patients over an extended period, and to some extent derived from the example of King Lear's "abdication" and his search for confirmation of his value from his daughters as a situation driving perplexity and verbosity. In contrast to the typical interventions, I formulated the witnessing of the Fool in the play as a figure for bringing to view the focus on the person in the relation to Lear and to his life as a father and a king in ways that obscured other relations to desperate conditions, thus inviting us to rethink the situation as making researchable ways of navigating the tension between care as witnessing and as managerial.

The difficulty of sustaining the posture of witnessing under such conditions, noted in the figure of the Fool and his relationship to Lear, dramatizes the import of being partial to the particularity of the speech of dementia by grasping its revelations as if a narrative of a (second) story about the specificity of its relationship to mortality through the content of the verbiage it produces. The personal impressions that caregiving elicits and tries to "read" in the repertoire of dementia can arrest analysis unless used *allegorically* as a symptom, as a mark of the experience of the inevitability of death in the present *hic et nunc* that is forced upon the caregiver as a matter to witness. Being partial to the particularity of the other makes reference to the readiness to listen to such a melancholy lament on the end-of-life to and for this other and with this other at this time.

Bearing Witness

> Let us try to probe a little bit the notion of bearing witness. Is bearing witness purely and simply communication, too? Surely not. It's clear however that everything we attach value to as communication is of the order of bearing witness. Disinterested communication is ultimately only failed testimony, that is, something upon which everyone is agreed. Everyone knows that this is the ideal of the transmission of knowledge. The entire system of thought of

> the scientific community is based on the possibility of a communication that concludes with an experiment that everybody can agree on. The very institution of the experiment is a function of testimony. Here we are dealing with another sort of otherness.
>
> (Lacan [1955–1956] 1997, 38–39)

In this sense, it seems that the stigmatization of dementia sufferers that contemporary research on patient-centered care tries to correct might miss the real cause of alienation, by assuming it to be a function of depersonalized care that needs to be redeemed by formats that counsel dignity or respect for personal characteristics. Yet, such a conception of the sufferer as subject to stress seems to avoid rather than engage the person, because the anxiety of stressful relations to a condition is derivative, in contrast to the anxiety that enters into the formation of this symptom. In resisting a stimulus-response model of illness causing stress (body causing mind), we can rethink the formation of the symptom where some primordial stress in relation to historical conditions set the process in motion (and it would be a gloss of such a primary scene to describe it as "stress"). That is, the reputed anxiety in stress is not the primary anxiety or the "real" object (Blum 2011, 202–203, 222–223, 248–249).

In this chapter, I have suggested that such an orientation can rethink molecular idealism *and* its supposed transgression as formats that block our capacity to apprehend the intuitions of morality that are suffered and implicitly expressed. This method of social inquiry then always invites analysis rather than argumentative confirmation or rebuttal based upon evidence that is governed by the formulaic approaches (Blum and McHugh 1984). For example, in terms of an operational grasp, we move closer to a connection to the person when we begin to develop some sense of the ways in which the dementia is a manner of working-through desperation that is not simply a response to the stress of neurological deterioration. So we might ask, what is the desperation that dementia covers over in its word salad?

The Social Situation of Dying

The model of transmission rules the situation of counselling the Alzheimer's caregiver, whether family or professional, first, about how to respond to the apparently bizarre behavior by not finding its accusations and ravings "personal," but typically to be a function of brain deterioration, cognitive impairment and the like. Yet what remains unanalyzed, and a crucial source of resistance for all parties in this relationship, is the need to represent the experience of the inevitability of mortality and of the loss about which it must speculate.

Thus, the intersubjectivity of aging and death has extraordinary complications that are necessary to grasp as a feature of the care given. It is recognized that caregivers need to understand the situation of dementia, how to speak to the old and the dying and (if an outsider) to their families. If they do (as typically they must) token talk that is often viewed by the patient as obligatory (because the living are viewed as disengaged from the old and dying who tend to see themselves as burdensome in this state), then caregivers cannot change this situation, but need to be aware of how they are treated and oriented to, for example, as if they are managing the subject, or are unloving, opportunistic, or simply dutiful. We note how this dialectic of caregiving involves radical role reversals: just as the old and dying must relinquish previous independence and sovereignty, the family caregiver has typically to relinquish prior dependency, revealing in such a situation a Lear effect (from *King Lear* and the work of other theorists such as Cavell 1995) where abdication from life and the testing of relationships between one another constitutes the materials for hallucinations and transferences (the relation of abdication—from life—and madness typically unfathomable to the living even if intimate). Thus, the tendency of medical practice to treat dementia as a deteriorating cognitive function, even if credible in many cases, forecloses the opportunity to explore the subject status of both paranoia and helplessness on the one hand, and guilt and helplessness on the other, as ways of dealing with self vis-à-vis life and death.

If the idea of the "end-of-life" has weight as a phenomenological experience to which we orient, rather than as an indifferent mark, then the experience of impending death and its inevitability should be part of the speech and conduct of such a subject, even indirectly as part of the "text" of the subject, even in ways of which one might be unaware. In this respect, caregivers would need to track such implications by learning to read and hear the talk for such overtones. In this sense, we might learn not simply from psychology or any science of the mind, but from the analysis of texts and narratives as well, fully attuned to the idea that any such talk by people suffering dementia is talk that needs to be reflected upon as a text of sorts and with the same methods in use historically for approaching any text. Even before we might prejudge such talk as psychotic it is important to develop methods and procedures for approaching the representations as material for analysis. If the conventions of analysis have bequeathed to us such methods, then they have also provided access with images of the figuration at work in stories, not only with reference to "external" matters of facts, but to the doubling that any text does as it uses the materials at hand to speak of many other matters, say, metaphorically, analogically, or even allegorically. Following Benjamin ([1936] 1968), many have rescued allegory from its status as disreputable fable to seeing it as a method that attends to relations between different elements in the text.

Here is an example of how a conventional British scholar discovers the allegorical element in a fragment of text from Parmenides, the great Greek pre-Socratic philosopher:

> But Parmenides is plainly allegorizing. The allegory may of course be based on something akin to a mystical experience, but it is none the less an allegory… . Parmenides is not giving the literal record of a spiritual adventure but clothing his search for truth in an allegorical dress. Parmenides' poem may be called allegorical because it has two meanings—the superficial meaning which tells a story and the implied meaning which gives the essential

> message of the poet. He tells of a chariot journey through gates to a goddess, but what he really describes is the transition from ignorance to knowledge.
> (Bowra 1953, 39)

So here, the idea of "two meanings" in a text stamp it as allegorical in a way that denigrates the "superficial meaning" in contrast to the meaning that is essential. Of course, this assumes everything we need to explore, but in its way it does accredit the two-sidedness of the text, one side as shallow (surface) and the other as deep (essential), in ways we have come to ratify through distinctions such as content (shallow) and form (deep), or content (deep, substantive) and form (shallow, abstract), or speech (shallow) and language (deep). Benjamin translates this distinction in terms of the difference between symbol and allegory, or what Lacan would come to call the relation of symbolic order to the imaginary. Even better, Jacques-Alain Miller (1991) has translated these "two sides" as the relation of the overt story to the secret story, and the distinction can be made to resonate with a range of contrasts of levels in a text from competence and performance to manifest and latent dimensions of a dream.

Be aware, though, that we are not resurrecting anything but a renewed respect for the coexistence of stories on the surface (in Hegel's idiom) as undeveloped, implicit, and abstract (empty, as Lacan would say), "hidden" only by virtue of the way the formula (the signifying situation) possesses an automated familiarity (in the idiom of Wittgenstein), or of being seen-but-unnoticed (in the way of ethnomethodology). The mystery that allegory addresses in this way is not pursued by plumbing depths, but by working-through the unstated resonances held in abeyance by the formula. So the interlocutor to allegory would not be "literal," of course, in the way Bowra's description affirms, nor even symbolic, nor the manifest, but what we can imagine for the inquirer as inertia in contrast to development. That is, the allegorical begins to identify a relationship to material that seeks to develop some matter lost to view and yet present as (what Benjamin calls) a "darkened horizon." Bowra speaks of "clothing" or "allegorical dress" in ways that lead us to appreciate the speaker as desiring to express some essential "message" in clothing or dress that could tempt us to treat this garb as what is essential, rather than the concealed message. Yet the speaker seems to clothe the speech as such because of the impossibility of putting into words the essential message, not from maliciousness or perversity, but because what is essential cannot be put into words. What cannot be put into words is not hidden from the words, but concealed in the words themselves.

Abdication

What was Lear doing when in abdicating his throne he offered to divide it among his three daughters, and how does this relate to dementia? If we understand, in this case, "abdication" as a figure for resignation from life, we can take it that Lear was dying and that the madness he displayed was in some way connected to his intuition of mortality. Note that it was not the fact of dying that produced the dementia but his relationship to his daughters and their reactions to his proposal.

What he proposed was that whosoever could demonstrate their love for him would win this inheritance. The intersubjective relation, his reaction to their reactions, produced or "caused" the madness. Why?

As one facing death and exercised by the question of his value in life as marked by his value for them, as a father, he sought confirmation as a sign of his value, a sign that could confirm their recognition of him as one of value. Lear wanted confirmation of his value as a father and for his life led from his daughters. To elicit such recognition, he offered to bribe them if they could demonstrate in words the love for him that he needed to hear. Since he needed to hear that he was of value, and to recognize in this a sign of the value of his life, the possibility of his appearing otherwise as a father and a man must have been at stake. In other words, the question of the value of a life is an open question, perhaps most poignant upon impending abdication, because the attachment of parent to child is overdetermined, a result of many influences. If they do love him it could be a lie, due only to his position and not to his person, and then they do not love him but love that (other) part of him; then again, they might love him because he is their father, loving the father in him (or the duty to love a father) and not loving him in particular.

As Cavell (1995) reiterates in his discussion, what Lear recognizes in the responses of others, and particularly Cordelia's reaction to his demand, is the violation of their intimacy, and so, is another sign of the disavowal of love for which he is now asking. This quest as such, mirrors his desire to obtain such reassurance in a way that can only reveal himself to himself as both undeserving of love that he had never given, and as a man who desperately needs to commemorate what he had never been able to give, love, and what he had never recognized in himself as one whose life was ruled by such disavowal. Lear, as any one, must face up to the possibility that he was a non-lover, that is, that he is and will be recalled as a non-lover despite his protestations.

Here, the abstraction of the parental function, and in this guise as the paternal function, can only be illuminated in the flash of the bribe as a mirror of his otherness, the two parts of the man that had never come together. That Cordelia could not tell him what he wants to hear reveals to him his blindness towards their intimacy as if in making it public he forfeits any claim upon it, being led to misrecognize the false love of the sisters as true and the true love of intimacy (and Cordelia) as false. What I am suggesting is that the play permits us to recognize the possibility that madness as a text of hallucination is the demented soliloquy of one sharing with a witness, the desire to be confirmed in life as mattering, as significant. In this sense, we must tread carefully in assuming the fundamental incoherence of age-related dementia unless we begin to develop methods for reading and formulating such a text. Baudelaire captures this potential for hallucination to make reference to another story.

> Imagination is not fantasy … imagination is an almost divine faculty which perceives … the intimate and secret relations of things, the correspondences and the analogies.
>
> ("Notes on Poe," quoted in Benjamin [1927–1940] 1999, 285)

This invites further analysis around, for example, the connection of the text of hallucination to the desire to articulate the experience of nihilism in an idiom that could appear both poetic and mad. Such analysis could take up Baudelaire's invitation to explore the imaginative character of the "intimate and secret" experience of end-of-life and its apparent incoherence. This research is underway.

Conclusion

The brain is a formula that we have engaged, and so, the locus of a discourse that remains essentially problematic. Here, then, it is not a matter of whether physical decline *is* essential to aging, since it must always remain an important factor, but rather how the actor orients to such a condition as needing to be grounded. The governing relationship posited here depends upon seeing the brain as the crucial mediator in "causing" physical decline and any acute disintegration, but the sacred character of such a profane illustration invariably invites working-through. In this sense, it is the truth of the convention (of the formula that stipulates the causal agency of the brain as what is essential) that must be oriented to as a beginning distinction that has to be grounded interpretively and for which some demonstration is required. What is always "worked-through" is the inflexibility of the convention, in part by engaging the unthought implications it masks in the way such "work" is much like the intervention in the common speech or orthodoxa. We have begun to disclose how the enthusiasm over the elegance and causal precedence of the brain in human affairs functions as reverie, piety, and reassurance for beleaguered mortals.

References

Baudrillard, Jean. (1977 and 1981) 1983. *Simulations*. Edited by Sylvère Lotringer. Translated by Paul Foss, Paul Patton, and Phil Beitchman. New York: Semiotexte.

Benjamin, Walter. (1927–1940) 1999. *The Arcades Project*. Edited by Rolf Tiedemann. Translated by Howard Eiland and Kevin McLaughlin. Cambridge, MA: Belknap Press of Harvard University Press.

——. (1936) 1968. "The Storyteller: Reflections on the Works of Nikolai Leskov." In *Illuminations: Essays and Reflections*, edited by Hannah Arendt, translated by Harry Zohn, 83–110. New York: Schocken Books.

Bielski, Zosia. 2010. "Dementia Risk Higher for Spouses of Sufferers." *The Globe and Mail*, May 6. Available at: www.theglobeandmail.com/life/health/dementia-risk-higher-for-spouses-of-sufferers/article1559465/. Last accessed October 27, 2013.

Blum, Alan. 2011. *The Grey Zone of Health and Illness*. Bristol: Intellect Press.

Blum, Alan and Peter McHugh. 1984. *Self-Reflection in the Arts and Sciences*. Atlantic Highlands, NJ: Humanities Press.

Bowra, C. M. 1953. *Problems in Greek Poetry*. Oxford: Clarendon Press.

Brooker, Dawn. 2003. "What is Person-Centred Care in Dementia?" *Reviews in Clinical Gerontology* 13 (3): 215–222.

Burke, Kenneth. 1957. *The Philosophy of Literary Form: Studies in Symbolic Action*. Berkeley, CA: University of California Press.

Cavell, Stanley. 1995. "Emerson's Constitutional Amending: Reading 'Fate.'" In *Philosophical Passages: Wittgenstein, Emerson, Austin, Derrida*, 12–41. Cambridge, MA: Blackwell.

Cottrell, V. and R. Schulz. 1993. "The Perspective of the Patient with Alzheimer's Disease: A Neglected Dimension of Dementia Research." *The Gerontologist* 33 (2): 205–211.

Freud, Sigmund. (1895) 1957. "Mourning and Melancholia." In *Volume 11, On Metapsychology: The Theory of Psychoanalysis*, translated by James Strachey, 245–268. London: Penguin.

Galvin, J. E., J.E. Duda, D.I. Kaufer, C.F. Lippa, A. Taylor, and S.H. Zarit. 2010. "Lewy Body Dementia: Caregiver Burden and Unmet Needs." *Alzheimer Disease and Associated Disorders* 24 (2): 177–181.

Garfinkel, Harold. 1967. *Studies in Ethnomethodology*. Englewood Cliffs, NJ: Prentice Hall.

Iemolo, Francesco, Giovanni Duro, Claudia Rizzo, Laura Castiglia, Vladimir Hachinski, and Calogero Caruso. 2009. "Pathophysiology of Vascular Dementia." *Immunity & Ageing* 6 (13): 1–9.

Kitwood, Tom. 1997. *Dementia Reconsidered: The Person Comes First*. Buckingham: Open University Press.

Kolata, Gina. 2010. "In Spinal Test, Early Warning on Alzheimer's." *New York Times*, August 10. Available at: http://query.nytimes.com/gst/fullpage.html?res=9C02EFD816 39F933A2575BC0A9669D8B63&pagewanted=all. Last accessed October 27, 2013.

Kontos, Pia C. 2006. "Embodied Selfhood: An Ethnographic Exploration of Alzheimer's Disease." In *Thinking About Dementia: Culture, Loss, and the Anthropology of Senility*, edited by Annette Leibing and Lawrence Cohen, 195–217. Piscataway, NJ: Rutgers University Press.

Kontos, Pia C. and Gary Naglie. 2007. "Bridging Theory and Practice: Imagination, the Body, and Person-Centred Dementia Care." *Dementia: The International Journal of Social Research and Practice* 6 (4): 549–69.

Lacan, Jacques. (1955–1956) 1997. *The Seminar of Jacques Lacan, Book III: The Psychoses 1955–1956*. Edited by Jacques-Alain Miller. Translated by Russell Grigg. New York: Norton.

McLuhan, Marshall. 1964. *Understanding Media: The Extensions of Man*. Toronto: McGraw Hill.

Miller, Jacques-Alain. 1991. "Reflections on the Formal Envelope of the Symptom." Translated by Jorge Jàuregui. *lacanian ink* 4: 13–22.

Mittleman, M.S., D.L. Roth, D.W. Coon, and W.E. Haley. 2004. "Sustained Benefit of Supportive Intervention for Depressive Symptoms in Caregivers of Patients with Alzheimer's Disease." *American Journal of Psychiatry* 161 (5): 850–856.

Quenqua, Douglas. 2011. "Rethinking Addiction's Roots, and Its Treatment." *New York Times*, July 10. Available at: www.nytimes.com/2011/07/11/health/11addictions.html. Last accessed July 20, 2011.

Schroeder, Steven, Marcus Krupp, Lawrence Tierney, and Stephen McPhee. 1990. *Current Medical Diagnosis and Treatment*. Norwalk (CT): Appleton and Lange. Cited in Kontos 2006.

Schutz, Alfred. (1953) 1973. "Common Sense and Scientific Interpretation." In *Collected Papers, Volume 1: The Problem of Social Reality*, edited by Maurice A. Natanson, 7–34. The Hague: Martinus Nijhoff.

Thomas. W. I. and D.S. Thomas. 1928. *The Child in America: Behavior Problems and Programs*. New York: Knopf.

Weber, Max. (1921–1922) 1947. *The Theory of Social and Economic Organization.* Translated by A.M. Henderson and Talcott Parsons. New York: The Free Press.

Wittgenstein, Ludwig. (1953) 1958. *Philosophical Investigations.* Edited by G.E.M. Anscombe and R. Rhees. Translated by G.E.M. Anscombe. New York: Macmillan.

8 The Writing Machine — Public Health, Dementia, and the Spell of the Brain as an Object of Social Enthusiasm

Introduction

Descriptions of public health advice as a body of knowledge can be straightforward in the mode of observations of health campaigns or programs influenced by models of knowledge transfer that are directed to facilitate the reception of such information. Attempts at more critical analyses can be done by presuming to unmask ideological presuppositions of health information (for example, idols of medicalization, expertise, or avaricious pharmaceutical agents), and/or as disclosing dependencies on conventions in the manner of descriptions of popular culture and its stereotypes (for example, exposure of assumptions of stigma). Despite the force of such a range of approaches, some conception of the social form of information as an object of desire within the context of a symbolic order is typically an uncounted part in such descriptions. This work has been prepared in part through Debord's (1994) conception of spectacle, Baudrillard's (1990) distinction between fascination and seduction, and Benjamin's (1999) notion of the enthusiasm as a turning point that Foucault developed, and has appeared in the works of others such as Lacan. I will intervene in this discourse in order to work-through an analysis of the social form of an enthusiasm with particular reference to the relationship integral to the collective fascination with neurology.

One way to treat medicine as a cultural phenomenon is to resist its sacralization as anything more than a phenomenon of the symbolic order so that we can begin to analyze the way its powerful and compelling information functions as normatively coded. In this sense, socially constructed elements of standards and the ambiguous implications of interdictions invariably enter into the formation of a self. By virtue of this, the demands upon such a self are also capable of stimulating fear, anxiety, and guilt with respect to prescribed courses of action.[1]

What is legitimized in this way is the corpus of information that anyone and everyone is expected to acquire and that is presumed to constitute adequate knowledge of the well-informed citizen (Schutz 1946). More than this, though, information often functions to center a degree of fascination with respect to its need to be absorbed or digested and the perils of inaction that can become phobic (Plamper and Lazier 2010). Particularly in the case of health care, the pundit can be viewed as a social type that reminds and alerts members of the dangers of being uninformed or of being inactive with respect to what they should know.

Society Represents Itself

I use Durkheim's conception of society as a writing machine that displays itself in the images and representations circulating in its environment as a collection of intimations and indications that are "inference rich." In this way, a society can be seen as presenting itself in signs that are implicitly legible on the surface of a text that can either be the start of a movement toward deciphering or accepted and laid to rest as if self-evident. Mike Gane (1983) suggests that for Durkheim, such a writing is aptly represented in formats that condense and displace knowledge in different ways (its scripts, formulae, conventions, distinctions) that give body to the unstated but evocative knowledge of a collective, transforming conceptions as if the materialization of a code.

> [D]iscourse is marked by the appearance of formulae, of secular and sacred and political kinds, which condense social knowledge. They are characterized by all the attributes of social facts but particularly by objectivity and externality, and, [Durkheim] notes, by the fact that as codes their existence is separate from their application.
>
> (Gane 1983, 9)

The conception of a writing machine posits a collective as making itself observable in a textual fabric that can be read as mirroring ideals, standards, and objectives as if a dreamwork with layered meanings modeled after a primary process that penetrates and exceeds the surface indications. As Michael North (1994, 142) has stated, this assumption that language is the "surest representation of a people to itself" permits us to formulate language in a more robust way than lexical. This fabric identifies a social text inclusive enough to make reference to argot, clichés, slang, vernacular expressions, and music, including lyrics, titles, song titles, and gestures and inflections of all sorts. Though neither Gane nor Durkheim speak of a primary process, I suggest that the notion of the writing machine brings to view the resources Freud used to analyze the formation of the dream and its "work" as the materialization of a symbolic order.

At the most immediate level, such writing makes reference to the images in circulation when we understand imagery as representations oriented to as usages that can be "read" as signifiers to engage. In this sense, any environment is legible as an inherited body of images, and so, "reading" an environment is not an abstract exercise but part of an ongoing relationship to conditions that take shape in conventions that seem external and coercive, as Durkheim says, and appear as grounds of inference and action in their being oriented to and engaged. Thus, the writing machine is more than literary in the way connotations and implications of many kinds can be oriented to as grounds of inference. Alfred Schutz has written on the ways such signs, symbols, marks, or cues can serve as "data" in everyday life. Further, in Baudelaire's sense, such "writing" includes any usage that can be oriented to as a display of the "look" of a society. For example, adverts in the media and in all visual representations can be read to see how pleasure is represented in scenes of action and activity.

This means that the notion of a writing machine applies not only to information conveyed in news or stories and formats of various kinds, but to connotations evoked by visual images in examples such as Sunday supplements, fashion, decoration and design, cinema, signage, the built environment, and the appearance of persons and things including doors, windows, or furniture, and any indications that are legible in some sense. This includes, of course, literary indices ranging from fiction to documents of various kinds, to laws, policies, legal edicts and descriptions and resolutions in cases, but also complaints in the media, opinions of all sorts and on all media, lyrics and refrains, statistical inventories, even budgets, graphic displays, and cues, clues, and signs of every sort including expressions. For example, legal cases where interpretation around issues in selected situations show different kinds of appeals or excuse, different accounts, and the like with respect to motivation, guilt, and so on, can convey images of conduct and of alternative actions and their appraisal that are used to typify situations.

Information, for example, is no different in this respect, not simply because its factual status is constructed, but because the relevance and urgency with which it is invested as such an edited phenomenon always reveals assumptions about the differences that it claims to make for those to whom it is directed. Thus, the news not only affirms the value of objectivity often noted but the format of the 6 o'clock or 11 o'clock news show informs us about the daily rhythms and priorities of a collective and its scheduling, conceptions of concentration and attention, and of what is noteworthy or of no matter, in the way all programming makes statements implicitly about the orientation of the audience and must theorize in ways that regulate its expectations about the audience and the "success" of its products. Durkheim uses the metaphor of the writing machine not simply to debunk ideologies and to note the fact of pervasive and inescapable social construction, but to identify an ever-present source of data that is accessible for studying the "inference rich" interpretive infrastructure we might imagine to implicitly bind a collective (Durkheim 1933).

In the present case this leads us to examine public health discourse as information that evokes concerted and implicit conceptions of the relation of mind to body and of well-being and its limits and possible infractions. We can call such writing a machine to emphasize its systemic character as a normative order guided by conceptions that idealize objectives, processes, and mechanisms of association, but more specifically, because such an order seems to have an automated character that discloses it as an apparatus governed by impersonal factors. How a system can be both normative (and an upshot of what seems like "personal" or subjective orientations) and automated (and what seems like a rule-governed or impersonal mode of operation) is precisely a question that the notion of a writing machine raises for Durkheim, that is, the question of the tension between its freedom and constraint, or its character as both profane and sacred. In this way automation makes reference to the untouchable ambiguity that remains unspoken in any collective while profanity refers to the ordering of normative elections that seem ostensibly to regulate the order (Blum 2014).

Yet the notion of the writing machine makes reference to more than the automated character of a normative order (or what scientists call a complex system) but to the way in which the writing of a collective is transformed into a machine from its original status as a tool. The writing machine, much like a mimesis of the movement of routinization from charisma to bureaucracy that Weber identified, exemplifies the movement toward standardization noted in all collective pursuits. The writing machine, then, is a sociological cliché that notes the inevitable standardization that any symbolic order must undergo, revealing the "system" expressed in its generalized other as a normative order and its intimation of excess or of a connotative surplus rooted in fundamental ambiguity ("values") that it holds in abeyance.

The Cliché

A good example of the action of the writing machine is the cliché whose standardization is both evocative and a beginning for critique. Analysis of the cliché shows that its routine condemnation for triteness conceals its function in many different textual strategies (Amossy 1982). In one sense, the cliché can function as a posit that standardizes differences among users by establishing a provisional locus of agreement from which discussion can proceed: in this process, the discussion moves not away from the posited agreement but returns toward it to reformulate it and its unspoken legacy (see the methodical movement of writing as revision in McHugh *et al.* 1974). In this sense the cliché shows the two-sided ambiguity of the posit that begins discussion as a resource *and* serves as the focus of its topicalization, combining both functions in its usage as a mark of fundamental ambiguity. The best example of this status of the cliché as a posit is the case of improvisational theater in which the commonplace is used as a starting point or "opener" for discussion that proceeds by moving on in ways that reformulate this beginning. We posed this as the problem of writing as revising in *On the Beginning of Social Inquiry* (McHugh *et al.* 1974) and I develop this further (Raffel and Sandywell, 2016). Even dementia or any diagnostic category is like this for us, serving as the image of a relationship upon which we might settle for beginning to speak together *and* as the usage that our common speech engages as the content for its analysis.

We note that if the cliché is the material form of the standardization suggested by the notion (and cliché) of the writing machine, then the relationship to the cliché as either/or compliant and passive or engaged and critical connects easily to the conception of habit. Durkheim (1961, 262, 264) speaks of the existence of the "collective habit" as coexisting in its way as a feeling of regularity, showing how self-consciousness takes stereotypical form (Gane 1983, 18) as a kind of social framework that condenses and displaces diversity in homogeneous formulae (see also Raffel, 1979).

If habituation depicts a passive relationship to the cliché, then this passivity does not necessarily mean resignation or complacency, but a desire to accept its usage provisionally as a starting point for "working-through" or the *durcharbeiten* that Freud (1958) called analysis. In this sense of passivity, habituation makes reference to the comatose of the speaker (see Socrates' example in *The Republic*) who repeats the formula mechanically instead of engaging it as the beginning for an imagined trajectory of the action of inquiry. A more active alternative sense of habituation does not simply repeat the lore concerning dementia, but uses what it knows about dementia to begin to unsettle this knowledge that it shares by reflecting upon the bond cemented by the cliché. Unsettling the usage or challenging habituation in this sense is then a beginning toward unloosening the hold of the formula upon oneself as a way of breaking the habit of the speech. Yet, if the liberation promised by such a challenge reveals the cliché at first as a tool for uprooting the hold of language upon its subject, then the demands of speaking together can only disclose automation as the ever-present environment for mutually oriented social action.

The Conception of an Enthusiasm

It is in this way that public health can begin to appear not simply as a display of information on governing our bodies ("all the news that's fit to print") but as an interpretive structure bordering areas such as mass media and popular culture, communication, information and "knowledge" transfer, and relations of science and/or medicine to society. As such, this writing of society in its heterogeneous voices can highlight tensions and contradictions that render the discourse as a whole problematic in every respect. Perhaps the crucial tension in such a writing concerns who has the authority to enforce interpretive control, particularly in the exchanges between expertise and its backing and support, lay opinion, and the status of evidence, all of this in relation to the question of what is worth believing.

I analyze the collective engagement with the disease known as Alzheimer's and the dementia reputed of it as an almost addictive dependency upon socially standardized formulae that attribute causal agency to the brain in the absence of clinching evidence. I view this gesture of honoring the brain as an expression of a collective struggle for self-knowledge in the face of what must remain unknown and threatens to leave us paralyzed, in particular, intuitions regarding the enigma of aging and its relations to death and the inevitability of loss in life that always threatens to extinguish our sense of an eternal present and invites us to reaffirm our commitment to any present as a collective need and desire. In this sense, the engagement with age-related dementia can be seen as a social phenomenon and not simply as a medical "fact." This follows from a method for exploring any and all conceptions of public health as part of a structure of interpretations or symbolic order that relates to medical views and public policies as part of an organization of knowledge and its discursive possibilities.

The Biomedical Revolution

In this way, I begin by treating public health, in part, as what is called popular culture as standard and formulaic talk and work-through that usage. Such a discourse structures (legitimates) expectations regarding health and illness and the administration of care and the views of those ruled by such notions. Parallel to the ways in which Foucault discussed the French Revolution as an icon of modern life, oriented to and engaged as a spectacle, I focus upon how age-related dementia in Alzheimer's disease and the neurological reasoning that frames the problem is engaged as such a spectacle, constituting a popular enthusiasm amenable to analysis.

> What is significant is not the exploits and gesticulations of the revolutionary drama itself … [but] the way in which the Revolution exists as spectacle, the way in which it is greeted everywhere by spectators who are not participants but observers, witnesses, and who, for better or worse, let themselves be caught up in it … What is significant is the enthusiasm for the Revolution.
>
> (Foucault 1984, 17–18)

Foucault's treatment of madness suggests the possibility that fascination with public health and with the brain as an enigmatic object is an analogous icon of modern life.

In its focus as an enthusiasm, the discourse of public health surrounding the example of dementia is much like what sociology has identified as a fad, or craze, that grips populations in the way of any riveting fixation. Note that this observation does not disqualify the empirical status of the phenomenon, for the fact of dementia might be as certain as the fact of the French Revolution, invariably coming to view as a collective preoccupation and accessible for analysis in that guise. Further, as a social fact the analytic status of an enthusiasm does not necessarily connote pathological effects such as hysteria or phobia, though these similarities can raise suggestive questions regarding this border that separates an enthusiasm from such neighbors. One question to pose eventually is how the conversion of enthusiasm into spectacle then raises concerns for the pathological status of spectacle itself, as phobic, hysterical, or in some way destructive for the collective. It is this border and its demarcation that the pundit appropriates as territory for speculation in ways that we will consider later in the chapter. Health reporting and health news seem especially ripe for such punditry.

It is important to note that part of the structure of such enthusiasms is the idea of their timeliness, urgency, or occasion as a critical event that requires edification. In this way, the notion of the enthusiasm as marking a significant relation to knowledge is assumed to make necessary an urgent project for disseminating the best available information concerning the clarification of any and all problems it creates. To paraphrase Foucault here, what is significant is the "enthusiasm" for dementia and how spectators (who are not simply participants as Foucault says) get "caught up in it."

The grammar of the enthusiasm makes reference to features that allow us to differentiate it from neighboring figures of speech such as fad, spectacle, cultural stereotype, and the like, that members are always described as becoming attached to in fervent ways. In this chapter, the "object" of an enthusiasm seems to be the brain, but this is only the surface of the imaginative structure of what has been called biomedicine that seems to make possible the oriented and arrested fascination that Baudrillard (1983, 89) discussed in the case of cybernetics and its "molecular idealism." From this perspective, if biomedicine depicts a corpus of knowledge and implicitly idealizes a subject who is supposed to know (Lacan 2002), then enthusiasm begins to formulate the relationship of the subject of biomedicine to the knowledge he/she is supposed to know and the trials and tribulations that mark the complexity of this discourse. Yet, when the relationship to biomedicine becomes arrested, we still have to distinguish it from the fad, the craze, and even from the catastrophic preoccupation with the end of the world or with what has been called "ticking time bomb" scenarios. Here we can ask, just what seems to make the enthusiasm different? It is to Walter Benjamin and Foucault that we must turn.

> Definition of the "modern" as the new in the context of what has always already been there … There has never been an epoch that did not feel itself to be "modern" in the sense of eccentric, and did not believe itself to be standing directly before an abyss. The desperately clear consciousness of being in the middle of a crisis is something chronic in humanity. Every age unavoidably seems to itself a new age. The "modern" however, is as varied in its meaning as the different aspects of one and the same kaleidoscope.
>
> (Benjamin 1999, 544–5)

What is remarkable is that Benjamin unties the relation of modernity to industrialization, alienation, rationalization that have seemed the typical formulae, by revealing the connection of its overestimation of its present to something "chronic," the desire of every generation to dramatize its present as unprecedented, whether as moment of progress or crisis, in ways suggesting the affirmation of the present as a turning point. The modern, defined as an unreflective celebration of the present as turning point, seems to give itself meaning as a period with value, a time worth inhabiting and worthy of commitment that is more than doing time. In this way Benjamin hints at the condition as chronic because of its connection to time and mortality, that any present invests itself with value as being different in quality and not more of the same, by overestimating the drama and significance of its moment. Yet, if this overvaluing of itself is chronic, then how can Benjamin treat it as hell?

> The "modern," the time of hell. The punishments of hell are always the newest things going in this domain … What is at issue is … that precisely in that which is newest the face of the world never alters, that the newest remains, in every respect, the same. This constitutes the eternity of hell. To determine the totality of traits by which the "modern" is defined would be to represent hell.
>
> (544)

If the situation is chronic, then this is a normal social fact and not hell. What must be hell is other people as in Sartre's formula, the enthusiasts who in overvaluing their moment and its accomplishments in breathtaking reverence for its unprecedented character show not a lack of historical awareness or of academic refinement, but an inability to reflect upon their automated relation to their present and their need to accept its limits as the different façade of a face that remains the same. Escape from hell in Benjamin's sense would be akin to developing a relation to the structure of enthusiasm at any present and in this chapter I am using public health, molecular idealism, and neuromania as such an occasion. Yet, "escape" involves dissenting from declarations of our being condemned to hell, not by simply repeating an adversarial transference/counter-transference relationship to the enthusiasm or to the enthusiast as interlocutor, but by developing our resources to use the enthusiasm as an occasion for repositioning it as speech driven to sustain itself as worthwhile. In other words, the analysis of an enthusiasm should enable us to create a representation of the value that sustains it, the "ought" to which it answers (Simmel 2010).

Dementia is then a good example of the stimulating character of information, showing how it is capable of producing excitement of a different order from addictive pleasures or sensually engaging moments through its capacity to arouse the excitement of uncertainty over prospects and actions (Bielski 2010; Kolata 2010; Kontos 2006; Kontos and Naglie 2007). For example, to many, information about conspiracies, the end of the world, or even about its beginnings are truly exciting and capable of subjecting them to immersion in news concerning the events on which they inform. Part of this excitement (in the case of dementia) seems to be a feature of its inevitability as a correlate of aging, stimulated in this way by the unpredictability that such anticipation seems to encourage. Yet this only makes sense when we understand the excitement as linked not simply to the fact of the disease and its inevitability but to the call for action that it requires. In this sense, if what the enthusiasm reveals are the perils of inaction, what seems truly exciting might be the need to be responsive to this decision point, and the threat of inaction and its consequences that it brings to view. Can it be that such a macabre view of information discloses deliberation over inaction and its horrible consequences to be one way in which health science and its narratives give meaning to life (by keeping us involved, preoccupied, busy with thoughts of consequences of actions and inaction)?

The Status of a Collective Fixation

So, getting caught up in dementia, being swept away by its fascination in public life, most apparent in the mass media and pundits reporting on medical problems, is our phenomenon of interest as a start, our dependent variable, and to examine the structure of such fascination as a social and cultural phenomenon we explore a sample of the popular discourse in circulation. If the dependent variable then appears as "being swept away" that is displayed in representations of dementia (say, as epidemic, plague, or crisis), then the independent variable would be culture and the kinds of interpretive apparatus it brings to bear on conceptions of disease, aging, and mortality that are relevant to the specific case of dementia.

Note that an essential parameter of the grammar of public health as spectacle is the imperative call to action, the requirement that some form of remediation or intervention is necessary and desirable. This is the way in which the value of knowledge transfer is converted to the public health discourse through the action of preventative medicine and its various and sundry initiatives condensed in the figure of the campaign. This is important for grasping dementia as a spectacle of arresting urgency because its critical nature is viewed as demanding information to relieve the emergency, whether in the form of biomedical findings or self-help advice. I will first examine the ways in which the enthusiasm is constructed, publicized, and formulated in the popular media as an urgent matter of concern and as a body of information that needs to be translated and disseminated for the good of a population, and so, of collective value.

Disseminating Enthusiasm as Knowledge Transfer

In part, the contemporary landscape of health care inherits the Cartesian model for communicating knowledge as a one-dimensional top-down movement from producers to recipients, a site for anticipating improvement through enlightened informatics that flows in the way of transmission rather than translation.

In relation to the case of dementia, the same problem appears insofar as the main focus now seems to be directed to transmitting information, first, on the somatic sources of the disease in ways that anticipate making it intelligible to relevant sectors of the population, and then second, given such a foothold, disseminating recipes for dealing with such suffering in our midst, rules of thumb for coping with those who are afflicted. Typically, then, the knowledge to be passed on is both neurological and self-help, identifying as these extremes biomedical-inspired neurology and a cultural folklore typically treated as anecdotal: in the first, results are assumed as secure and trustworthy "findings," and in the second, as guides for handling uncertain situations that might be tried and tested in practice.

Popular Discourse

> Dementia is not a specific disease. It is a descriptive term for a collection of symptoms that can be caused by a number of disorders that affect the brain.
>
> (National Institute of Neurological Disorders and Strokes [NINDS] 2012, paragraph 6)

This reasonable opener recognizes the disease as a categorization aiming to collect and differentiate the phenomenon, identifying the causes as both multiple and limited to the brain. The correlation between the sign and the disease is always spurious in the absence of controls, a lesson that any elementary text in statistics and inference has long taught. The precedence of the body, then, based on problematic testimony of those dear to the afflicted who cannot make sense of the behavior shown, and of the speculative results of the autopsy, risk leaving anyone in a situation of anxiety where the brain seems to serve as a way of relieving and reducing the mystery surrounding abrupt and enigmatic reversals of behavior in an intimate who had been supposed to be otherwise (Schroeder, 2006).

It is this situation that we need to address by refocusing attention on the obscene aura of death that haunts the encounter in ways that might drive all touched to search for more satisfying accounts. In this respect, we need not simply accept the brain as an explanation for the symptom no matter how cogent the account seems, but query its place in this and related situations that animate the collective representation of health and illness and its surreptitious but vital link to the question of mortality. This is why reliance upon the medical research on dementia in Alzheimer's is less important for our purposes than an examination of the ways that the fears surrounding representations of dementia circulate and are digested in collective life as objects of anxiety.

That medical research in no way confirms the vernacular conception of dementia makes it only relevant to my inquiry as a symptom, as one of the voices in the collective writing and speaking about the phenomenon, and not to be treated as authoritative by virtue of its results. For example, note the absence of irony in the authoritarian hubris of the typical definition, its foreclosure of the question of the meaning of dementia.

> All forms of dementia result from the loss of nerve cells and/or the loss of communication among the cells. The human brain is a very complex and intricate machine and many factors can interfere with its functioning. Researchers have uncovered many of these factors, but they have not yet been able to fit these puzzle pieces together to form a complete picture of how dementia develops.
>
> (NINDS 2012, paragraph 6)

This encomium to the brain characterizes not only medical science but many areas, even in the humanities, that anticipate progress "right around the corner" (Žižek 1997) in the capacity of science to unravel the complexity of this mysterious ("intricate") machine, a machine so fascinating that researchers from all fields tend to find it beautiful or, as they might say, "awesome." Here, humans condemned to mortality still find elegant the machinery of their human brains, perhaps in the expectation that such a sublime mechanism will distract them from other concerns of matter (see Blum 2011b).

The Brain Causes an Epidemic

> Alzheimer's cases to soar in coming decades, say researchers while calling for national plan to deal with burden.
>
> The annual cost of dementia is projected to soar tenfold in the next generation, a stark illustration of the impact an aging Canadian population will have on the health-care system.

[…]

Dementia is just one of the chronic health conditions on the rise as the grey tsunami washes across the country. The number of seniors living with diabetes, heart disease, cancer, lung disease, and arthritis is also increasing.

Not only will looking after the aging population be financially costly—health already makes up more than 40 percent of government spending—but it will place a tremendous burden on the health and social services systems and, above all, families providing care to their loved ones.

"We need to get a lot smarter about how we deal with dementia," David Harvey, government relations officer at the Alzheimer Society of Canada, said in an interview. He noted that when people have dementia, they invariably have other health issues that complicate their care.

"If we don't take steps now to keep people out of long-term care, we will be spending a lot of money and place a crippling burden on families," he said.

The report, entitled "Rising Tide: The Impact of Dementia on Canadian Society," was commissioned by the Alzheimer Society and prepared by RiskAnalytica, a Toronto-based consultancy that specializes in risk management.

The report says that the country is facing a dementia epidemic and a "comprehensive national plan" is required to contain it.

(Picard 2010, paragraphs 1–2, 5–10)

We inquire into this form of talk, organized as it is around concerns for "rising costs" and the "burden" placed on services and caregivers, which does not query the condition of the "loved ones" themselves. It seems to be talk that treats the condition as self-evident to the author(ities), relevant only because of its "effects" upon costs and on those condemned to care for sufferers, which implicitly raises the question of who is the real object of suffering—society, caregiver, or afflicted one? Here, too, is the vision of a "rational plan" that might address both the rising costs and the emotional burdens, a plan sensitive to both economics and psychology as these are conventionally conceived. The voice of government in the guise of the policy specialist implicitly anoints itself as needed to coordinate efforts. Since the plan in a sense is created by the epidemic or crisis, it might be in the interest of planning, not out of malevolence but a surplus pleasure, to imagine crisis and epidemic everywhere, guaranteeing the importance of reports, pundits, and policy experts. This begins to suggest that noting the fact of epidemics and crises of all sorts, despite the medical pedigree of experts, might be part of a process that testifies to the production of public health as a social phenomenon, a phenomenon that invites inquiry of an altogether different kind (in the way that Marx famously said that among its effects and functions what crime produces are criminologists).

Thus, from a culturally oriented approach, setting up the problem of dementia requires intervening in the commentary that regards it as both plague and/or epidemic and a function of somatic incapacity that is assumed to be remedied by information on how the body functions and what persons need to learn in order to endure such contagious conduct. Contagion is implied by the fear of being exposed to dementia in caring for it, its deleterious effects appearing to cause depression. In this sense, the wave of concern for dementia in Alzheimer's disease and other reputed results of aging and its somatic deterioration exemplifies under the guise of a medical crisis the structure of public health as an imaginary relationship to the people and well-being. Despite the various kinds of epidemics, we can discern the similar grammatical structure, not intended to be an argument against medical and public health initiatives but an attempt to show how they work as part of a process, and though all of these activities are different, this analogical approach allows us to see some common mechanisms, for example, informed diagnosis rather than causal speculation gives ground for the intervention of expertise. Epidemic conveys the idea of a collectivity rather than the isolation of one victim with idiosyncratic character, and so, some vulnerability that might be impersonal in the sense of externally induced rather than an upshot of personal decision-making. Finally, the notion of danger suggests that steps need to be taken, preparation and pedagogy is required, because the phenomenon is both prevalent and invisible. Let me risk quoting myself here.

> The grammar seems to point first to the condition of a deceptive carrier, the difference between appearance and reality, and its detection by a qualified expertise. Secondly, the idea of epidemic suggests not merely that there are many of them but that they breed and so that there are common and perhaps incalculable conditions that nurture this collective in ways that can only proliferate and worsen unless remedial action is taken and some forceful authority is delegated to enforcement agencies with the rights to regulate this growth. Finally, reeducation is typically offered in the form of a curriculum proposing rules.
>
> (Blum 2011a, 179)

Dementia plays out the script of public health in specific ways. Firstly, if the very notion of epidemic dramatizes the danger of helpless and isolated persons in an anomic situation seeming to be ruled by contingency, then this effect is achieved by identifying the epidemic as collective rather than individual and, regardless of the variation in examples, assimilating all to the diagnostic category in ways that smooth out individual differences, disregarding any condition that is not amenable because it infers agency as a source of individual variation within the type. Secondly, to enforce this conception, the body and its structural continuity and discontinuity throughout a life is used as a normative standard for identifying an imaginary etiology of deterioration and decline, foreclosing the opportunity to introduce the history of the person, banning it as extraneous. And finally, this structural effect, treated as if an infection that is contagious, dramatizes the impersonality of the situation as a function both of the movement of the disease and its recruitment of targets, as an irrational flow that can only be neutralized through an appeal to expertise and the information this expertise might provide.

Benjamin tells us that the enthusiasm is a preoccupation of any modern moment with its modernity, with some sign (achievement, accomplishment) that reveals its time as a breakthrough and its present as if unprecedented. Therefore, the consumerist absorption in spectacle, and the rigidity in attachments to cultural stereotypes are not definitive for the enthusiasm because enthusiasm orients to its "object" as a sign of the unprecedented present and the significance of the present as an advance upon the past. In our case, the grammar of the enthusiasm can be specified as follows: by embodying in its project piety toward the brain and its "breakthrough" as a research object, the enthusiasm marks the present as a turning point that promises to demystify the enigma of human conduct, to provide new senses of agency and new conditions for action and change, and the prospect of a continuously malleable future "open" to constant productive achievements. Thus, the figure of turning point converts fascination through the Weberian notion of rationalizing the world into collective work of self-affirmation. The grammar of the enthusiasm emerges in relation to a conception of biomedical knowledge as a "turning point" that marks a decisive overcoming of past limitations. Apparently, the breakthrough for neurology in relation to age-related dementia is its claim to demystify the enigma of aging and its inevitable decline, allowing us to put aside or lay to rest whatever anxieties and concerns we might have. Enthusiasm for the conquest of such enigmas is the way our present congratulates itself on its unprecedented moment as a turning point. In this sense the enthusiasm adds to Weber's conception of demystification the sense of its status as a method for affirming the drive of life in each present. To do a Lacanian turn on Benjamin, the enthusiasm is a way of driving the dead life of any and every present to live again, to revitalize itself. The enthusiasm invests any present with life.

Expertise

One of the implications of the ways in which the health crisis is produced as plague, epidemic, or impending catastrophe, through the enthusiasm for remedial action that it always tries to mobilize with its information, is the creation of the figure of the pundit and his or her backing by bona fide research legitimated through medical data and, in this case, neurology. The pundit is anointed as one qualified to mediate between science and its constituencies by clarifying and representing the results of what is taken to be knowledge. The communicative situation is framed as an interaction or flow between such a pundit and a subject or consumer who is expected to receive and digest such a corpus of belief as adequate and bona fide (in ways that resonate with Lacan's question "what is the subject supposed to know?"). The pundit mediates between medical science in its neurological guise and the consumer (or caregiver) presumed to be in need of such advice in order to survive the situation. What the subject is supposed to know is whatever it will take to deal with the dementia sufferer in ways that appear to equate the goal of caregiving with the objective Alfred Schutz (1946) called for the "well-informed citizen." Yet the well-informed caregiver, whether through neurological information or self-help advice, is still prone to depression in ways that the mediation of information does not seem to eliminate. In fact, it is this limit that highlights the crisis, that it is not the absence of information and of its complete and perfect transmission that is the problem, but the fearful recognition that even the realization of this dream must leave a remainder.

In this sense, the most interesting facet of the dementia epidemic is not simply its social construction that has been noted by many (for example, Gubrium's [1986, especially 111–53]) exemplary treatment of public culture on how collective life brings to view examples of methods in use that describe and elaborate the symptoms, nor the way it might express a biomedical depersonalization of personhood (Kitwood 1997), but the way its interpretation as a cause of depression among caregivers tends to be treated as a result of burnout (the severe burdens of care) rather than as a reaction to the incomprehensible position of witnessing and awaiting the death of an intimate. The notion of burnout formulates the depression of the caregiver primarily as result of labor and of being overworked instead of seeing it as an upshot of the metaphysical angst of engaging the intuition of mortality. The solidarity between popular discourse and its neurological authorization supports this tendency to treat the caregiving relationship to dementia as a technical problem that can perhaps be survived through more and better information and self-help advice rather than being seen as the irreparable relationship between two witnesses to the poignancy of end-of-life and the limits of its meaningfulness as a matter to endure.

Enthusiasm and Contagion

The phenomenon of enthusiasm as the criterion of modernity simply confirms the manic dedication to productivity and progress since enthusiasm for the present presupposes a collective conception of the "now" as a departure from the past that is singular and unprecedented in its way. Further, the conception of enthusiasm reinforces the notion of progress and productivity by showing how only the subjectivity of people can be seen as standing in the way of the advance, and so is the only impediment, making subjectivity appear if a danger that requires regulation if progress is to occur. This is because the only obstacle to enthusiasm seems from this view to be a failure to recognize the singularity of the present moment and its opportune position in history for influence and consequential action. One feature of negativism appears as a failure to recognize this and to be enthusiastic as if resisting this view of advance. Yet negativism can also recognize the change and lament it as something other than an advance or as a moment of progress that has both positive and negative effects. Whether positive or negative, enthusiasm is needed to give each present moment a new lease on life by virtue of seeing it as consequential and capable of surpassing the past. Thus, if modernity is marked by enthusiasm as Benjamin suggests, this means that it sees the present at any time as a difference in kind from what precedes it by virtue of its unprecedented character as new in relation to what it surpasses. The hyperbole of such a relationship to the present is required by life itself in its effort to move ahead rather than stagnate and to mobilize the commitment and motivation to enhance and advance the inheritance that a present requires.

Different usages converge here in what Girard (1977) calls "mimetic contagion" to describe the contagiousness of the normative order in the way that norms must "infect" the subject through the idiom of stimulation that Lacan depicts as the imaginary. If norms stimulate the imaginary (in the way the environment "captures" the subject, in Lacan's idiom) this means that they limit and constrain the subject in a manner that can provide for adaptations of all kinds, including Freud's repression and forms of perversion and psychosis, as well as "legitimate" channels toward achievement and fulfillment. The contagiousness of the normative order suggests that it can embrace notions of both freedom and evil as Schelling noted, and that it can appear as a recurrent element of the modern psyche and its fluctuations, of longing and resignation, ecstasy and disappointment, invariably producing the range of observable modern anxieties and descriptions of stress and strain.

Moreover, Simmel's conception of the inevitable drive for self-transcendence (Lacan's jouissance) captures this dialectic between overstimulation, contagion, and infection "injected" by the normative order into its subject, always occasioning capacities for *eros* and *thymos* that can be positive or negative. That the "norms" can be engaged in many ways means that jouissance treads a thin line between compliance and excess as the subject invariably tries to administer a creative relationship to restraints (to rules, law, the generalized other, the distribution of the sensible) that appear at first to be inflexible and automated. Indeed, Simmel goes further here suggesting that it is not only norms and the order that stimulate excess but the limit itself insofar as the hole in the symbolic order makes observable to the subject the unknown that must persist as the remains. Thus, for Simmel it is not simply the normative that is provocative in establishing goals, objectives, interdictions, and the like, but the indeterminacy that remains or exceeds determination.

> One can never know another person absolutely, which would involve knowledge of every single thought and mood. Nevertheless, one forms some personal unity out of those fragments in which he alone is accessible to us.
> (2010, 309)

If the unknown (whether here of the other self, or to extend it, of oneself, and why not nature, too) is persistent and its perplexity a problem, it need not be paralyzing since it provides material for construction, invention, and improvisation. Simmel notes this when with reference to the inscrutable inner life of the individual he adds: "No other object can reveal or hide itself in the same way, because no other object modifies its behavior in view of the fact that it is recognized" (310). This very indefiniteness in the circulation of reciprocal knowledge, according to Simmel, makes the unknown a fertile source of improvisation as we mutually adapt to our ignorance in ways that are malleable and often creative.

If the unknown can be stimulating and an occasion to administer jouissance through the playful imagining of its meaning, it might also be voracious in its propensity to receive and digest material. Such material, stories, and information reveal how the writing machine works to make the unknown known, to make observable what cannot be seen, to make the invisible visible again. The writing machine tries to put the unknown into words. In the Simmelian sense that one can never know everything, we come face-to-face with the desire for stories and information, as a desire that the writing machine tries to satisfy, a desire for fiction and fact that can be moderate and/or extreme.

Story and Information

As Walter Benjamin (1968) says, the story contains something useful and makes possible the eventful exchange of experience whereas information tends to abbreviate. He says that the proverb is a ruin on the site of an old story. We can hear this as advice that the proverbial or commonplace is a "ruin" that conceals the story that time has threatened to extinguish (to kill) in a way that aligns the proverbial with the trace of a history, with memory that tries to regain what was lost. The proverbial begins in its way as witnessing that can make a place in memory and experience in the way listening leads to retelling. Witnessing occurs when life assumes transmissible form at point of death, anticipating the story and its ambiguity as surviving in the ways of material to rethink. He says that the name of the person serves as if an emblem, a marker for an untold story that gains in effectiveness if we disavow its literal detail and psychological shadings.

Thus, unlike the obituary or biography the story grips by its evocative power in ways that can be paradigmatic for the name of the one named, that is, instead of enumerating detail and chronology the name evokes as if a story, the name itself, much like the outer mark of the "inner sense" or spirit of whatever it names. In engaging the subject's hallucinatory speech as if such a story, we can now ask how this sign of dementia could be in its way in its very foreclosure of naturalistic and "psychological shadings" a way of making reference to a second story, a story of death.

> In the course of modern times dying has been pushed further and further out of the perceptual world of the living. . . . It turns out that this change is identical with the one that has diminished the communicability of experience to the same extent as the art of storytelling has declined.
>
> (Benjamin 1968, 93–94)

In other words the tendency to treat the name of a person as simple information or as a record of sorts rather than as the outer shape of an untold story, corresponds with the avoidance of death as a topic. According to Benjamin this is because death as the very topic of the story of a person and of the life behind the name is denied by treating the name as a mere record of information or as an archival trace, because the story of a person, when we truly listen, brings us face-to-face with the story of death.

> It is, however, characteristic that not only a man's knowledge or wisdom, but above all his real life—and this is the stuff stories are made of—first assumes transmissible form at the moment of his death. Just as a sequence of images is set in motion inside a man as his life comes to an end—unfolding the views of himself under which he has encountered himself without being aware of it—suddenly in his expressions and looks the unforgettable emerges and imparts to everything that concerned him that authority which even the poorest wretch in dying possesses for the living around him. This authority is at the very source of the story.
>
> (94)

Neither medicine nor caregiver can be expected to take pleasure in confronting this story of death. It should be more comforting to provide information on "the end-of-life" as a natural phenomenon including recipes of stress and pain relief for all parties. Witnessing though, asks the witness to make a place in their life for the retelling of the particular story as the story of particularity, in the gesture of a pledge, impossible but necessary almost as a safeguard against the ravages of time. This is the real indebtedness of the witness. This pledge disavows treating the name of the person as news, information, record, but as the experience of a relation that is passed on. What the pledge pledges is to make a place for the relationship in memory not merely through retelling its story as details and accomplishments, but by working through the placement of the life as such.

In contrast, the notion of news grounded in Schutz's conception of expertise or the pundit, focuses on its use of recipes as part of the desire to be well-informed that typifies a necessary adaptation to ignorance in relation to an inaccessible world that is always expressing itself nevertheless. The news pictures the world like the body that is always giving off information in gestures that can be "read" à la Goffman's approach to the signs emitted by the body. News brings the far near and allows us to develop a world picture of it for attaining (in principle) mastery. Self-knowledge can identify the imaginary of such comprehension as an objective of desire but the world picture or comprehensive mastery imagined for news as its "know-how" on how things work has always been differentiated from self-knowledge in important ways. In this sense, the story involves the loss of a singular experience for which excavation is required (see the journal, diary), which is how the story resonates with death and begins at the point of death (loss, decline), persisting as the ruin in Benjamin's usage (the proverbial) in the way of a hallucination at such a point. The proverbial intimates the remains or vestiges of a story and of an unfinished life (a life that has died but whose rethinking remains and so lives and is alive) whereas news finishes the life and makes it possible to avoid the sight of dying. The "explanation" offered by news lies in the connection of events not in the reader but in the events themselves for the reader. News desires to provide us with material for grounds of inference in the present by trying to relate action to the moment or future by revealing information as useful grounds of inference. The message of reproduction in news is that the finality of production (final cause, point, purpose) that Baudrillard says is lost in the series, i.e. the determinate conclusion that "I am what I say I am and I expect the same of you," suggests that our common bond in speaking together can only be maintained by excluding ambiguity as if our characterizations are both mutually oriented and self-evident as applicable to each in the same way.

Punditry

In his analysis of BS (bullshit) the philosopher Harry Frankfurt (2005) explores usage that could identify it with humbug or deceit as an invitation to mislead or with pretence or presumptuous self-presentation and resists such equivalences on the grounds that these are likely to be incidental or side effects of many practices. What seems essential to BS for Frankfurt is a tendency to orient to language in a way that is lax but where such irresponsibility is directed to the concept or signifier with a degree of indifference. This indifference toward language need not be deceitful and self-aggrandizing, but as he shows in his example of Wittgenstein's contempt for a friend's lazy expression, tends to exploit the ambiguity of the term not as a provocative response but as a way of avoiding working-through the usage.

Thus, as a relationship BS (and the bullshitter) is ruled by an apparent need for convenience in order to give pleasure in the speaking situation and to avoid exposing the complexity of the usage and how its ambiguity could qualify the notion of expertise. This is how the pundit can be said to produce empty talk or representations that inevitably need to be developed and are unformed, not simply because they are beginnings, but for the reason that they set themselves up as satisfying enough to be treated as ends, results, or as conclusive. Thus, the pundit impersonates well-informed talk not by lying but by stating the obvious as if its significance is grounded in a kind of expertise (presumed to be based on proximity or witnessing of an event or on access to specialized information).

BS is then not simply platitudinous but oriented toward taking an overview of the event in ways that choose to sacrifice engaging its complexity on the grounds that abbreviation is necessary and desirable for transmission (due to assumptions about the process or the recipient's limits), but really because the speaker has no resources or desire to engage the representation any further. The use of the overview as a format enables one to avoid trying to engage the ambiguity of the effort to put into words an inexpressible phenomenon. Frankfurt enables us to appreciate how punditry shows ways in which technical aspirations tend to diminish the weight of words and how the format of the news story, whether crime, politics, or health, is required to abbreviate what cannot be expressed and determined conveniently. Indeed, John Lanchester (2015) points out how much news is now automated and delegated to companies specializing in automating stories and reports. The tendency toward automated prose produced by the writing machine would suggest that death can only be represented in the format of externalized records, at best obituaries, and left, as a lived experience of the dying body, to representations in film, documentaries, the arts, and in particular, the novel.

Conclusion

In response to the automation of prose, historically, movements such as the automatic writing of Surrealism and all of the experimental initiatives out of France—such as the work of Perec and the Oulipo group, and the modernist innovations of Joyce, Woolf, and Faulkner—are well-known and discussed. In our contemporary climate the response to automated prose takes shape typically in the celebration of personal testimony as one example, attempting to show an alternative to biomedical depersonalization. But as Lacan points out, the testimonial assertion of the priority of the first-person voice treats affect as an end rather than beginning, avoids engaging resistances by calculating the anxiety to which the affect is a reply, and resists disrupting the sovereign grip of consciousness by holding fast to a model of symptom management rather than analysis. In this climate, theorizing is derided as "meta-talk" that turns its back on the immediate experience of a subject.

Of course, part of the writing machine today must include social media in all of its shapes as podcasts, chats, exchanges, rants and information processing, Instagrams, Facebook, blogging and the like, as usages that struggle with the desire for conversation under conditions of mechanical reproduction, a continuing source of data to be explored as a manifestation of the archive of orthodoxa. Under such conditions the writing machine performs at self-expression, offers of advice, simulations of expertise and criticality in ways intended to produce renewed senses of involvement and revitalization under conditions of alienation.

Between the extremes of biomedical reduction and such confessional affirmation, reflective thought risks losing its dialogical drive and its spirit for negation. In such an environment the question is always raised about best practices for offering challenges to conceptual formulae in the tepid linguistic marketplace. Among the best examples today are illustrated by the novels of David Markson that work to reformulate the writing machine in part as a collective archive ruled by a dialectic of free associations that constitutes the bits and pieces of any social inheritance as material to be engaged and collected, in the desire to rediscover problems that such fragments make possible (Markson, 1988). Care for our language involves contemplating and practicing the pursuit of different paths for unsettling the writing machine by revitalizing it and rescuing its visionary impulses in the aspiration to deliver us from its banality. Deleuze and Guattari (1987) have experimented with the pulse of writing in analyzing and reformulating Nathalie Sarraute's novels and theorizing on the viral movement in prose (Negrete, 2015). Perhaps we can best understand those who suffer extreme anxiety as engaged in this same struggle to find their voice in relation to the writing machine, those needing to poeticize their desperation. This invites us to develop a finely tuned ear for listening to what is beneath the surface rather than to continue prattling on, whether through the sanctimonious platitudes of punditry or the desultory support of intimates. As Wittgenstein, the Marx brothers, Scat, Joyce, Beckett, Anne Carson, and many others have confirmed, revolution just might begin in linguistic disruption rather than in the obsessive discourse of the university or its hysterical transgressive gestures, and the speech of dementia might very well be part of such an avant-garde.

Note

1 In this sense, such information, whatever its factual status, becomes an object of desire in collective life that binds and alienates, entering into what Parsons (1951, 24–68) famously called "pattern maintenance and tension release" among other functions (see also Parsons 1966, 11, for a synopsis where "legitimizing" is used to encompass all of the functions under culture).

References

Amossy, Ruth. 1982. "The Cliché in the Reading Process." Translated by Terese Lyons. *SubStance* 11 (2): 34–45.

Baudrillard, Jean. (1977 and 1981) 1983. *Simulations*. Edited by Sylvère Lotringer. Translated by Paul Foss, Paul Patton, and Phil Beitchman. New York: Semiotexte.

Baudrillard, Jean. 1990. *Seduction*. Translated by Brian Singer. New York: St. Martin's Press.

Benjamin, Walter. (1927–1940) 1999. *The Arcades Project*. Edited by Rolf Tiedemann. Translated by Howard Eiland and Kevin McLaughlin. Cambridge, MA: Belknap Press of Harvard University Press.

——. (1936) 1968. "The Storyteller: Reflections on the Works of Nikolai Leskov." In *Illuminations: Essays and Reflections*, edited by Hannah Arendt, translated by Harry Zohn, 83–110. New York: Schocken Books.

Bielski, Zosia. 2010. "Dementia Risk Higher for Spouses of Sufferers." *The Globe and Mail*, May 6. Available at: www.theglobeandmail.com/life/health/dementia-risk-higher-for-spouses-of-sufferers/article1559465/. Last accessed October 27, 2013.

Blum, Alan. 2011a. *The Grey Zone of Health and Illness*. Bristol: Intellect Press.

——. 2011b. "Life, Death and the In-Between: The Duck/Rabbit and the Face of the Clown." In *Spectacular Death: Interdisciplinary Perspectives on Mortality and (Un) representability*, edited by Tristanne Connolly, 21–41. Bristol: Intellect Press.

——. 2014. "Durkheim's Ruse: The Concept as Seduction." *Canadian Journal of Sociology* 39 (4): 567–594.

Debord, Guy. (1967) 1994. *The Society of the Spectacle*. Translated by Donald Nicholson-Smith. New York: Zone Books. Deleuze, Giles and Felix Guattari, 1987. *A Thousand Plateaux: Capitalism and Schizophrenia*. Minneapolis: University of Minnesota Press.

Durkheim, Émile. (1893) 1933. *The Division of Labor in Society*. Translated by George Simpson. New York: The Free Press.

——. (1912) 1961. *The Elementary Forms of the Religious Life*. Translated by Joseph Ward Swain. New York: Collier Books.

Foucault, Michel. 1984. "What is Enlightenment?" In *The Foucault Reader*, edited by Paul Rabinow, translated by Catherine Porter, 32–50. New York: Pantheon Books.

Frankfurt, Harry. 2005. *On Bullshit*. Princeton: Princeton University Press.

Freud, Sigmund. (1914) 1958. "Remembering, Repeating, and Working-Through: Further Recommendations on the Technique of Psychoanalysis II." In *Complete Psychological Works of Sigmund Freud, Vol. 12*, edited and translated by James Strachey, 145–168. London: Hogarth Press.

Gane, Mike. 1983. "Durkheim: The Sacred Language." *Economy and Society* 12 (1): 1–45.

Girard, René. (1972) 1977. *Violence and the Sacred*. Translated by Patrick Gregory. Baltimore: The Johns Hopkins University Press.

Gubrium, J.F. 1986. *Oldtimers and Alzheimer's: The Descriptive Organisation of Senility*. Greenwich, CT: JAI Press.

Kitwood, Tom. 1997. *Dementia Reconsidered: The Person Comes First*. Buckingham: Open University Press.

Kolata, Gina. 2010. "In Spinal Test, Early Warning on Alzheimer's." *New York Times*, August 10. Available at: http://query.nytimes.com/gst/fullpage.html?res=9C02EFD81639F933A2575BC0A9669D8B63&pagewanted=all. Last accessed October 27, 2013.

Kontos, Pia C. 2006. "Embodied Selfhood: An Ethnographic Exploration of Alzheimer's Disease." In *Thinking About Dementia: Culture, Loss, and the Anthropology of Senility*, edited by Annette Leibing and Lawrence Cohen, 195–217. Piscataway, NJ: Rutgers University Press.

Kontos, Pia C. and Gary Naglie. 2007. "Bridging Theory and Practice: Imagination, the Body, and Person-Centred Dementia Care." *Dementia: The International Journal of Social Research and Practice* 6 (4): 549–69.

Lacan, Jacques. 2002. "The Subversion of the Subject and the Dialectic of Desire in the Freudian Unconscious." In *Écrits: A Selection*, translated by Bruce Fink with Héloïse Fink and Russell Grigg, 281–312. New York. W.W. Norton & Company.

Lanchester, John. 2015. "The Robots Are Coming." *London Review of Books* 37 (5): 3–8.

Markson, David. 1988. *Wittgenstein's Mistress*. Champaign, Dublin: Dalkey Archive Press.

McHugh, Peter, Stanley Raffel, Daniel C. Fox, and Alan Blum. 1974. *On the Beginning of Social Inquiry*. London: Routledge and Kegan Paul.

National Institute of Neurological Disorders and Stroke. 2012. "Dementia: Hope Through Research." Available at: www.ninds.nih.gov/disorders/dementias/detail_dementia.htm?css=print. Last accessed February 15, 2013.

Negrete, Fernanda. 2015. "'A Vital Unliveable Force': Rhythm through Nathalie Sarraute and Schizoanalysis' Mosaic." *Mosaic* 48 (2): 83–98.

North, Michael. 1994. *The Dialect of Modernism: Race, Language and Twentieth-Century Literature*. Oxford: Oxford University Press.

Parsons, Talcott. 1951. *The Social System*. Glencoe, IL: The Free Press.

——. 1966. *Societies: Evolutionary and Comparative Perspectives*. Englewood Cliffs, NJ: Prentice-Hall.

Picard, André. 2010. "Costs to Soar as Aging Canadians Face Rising Tide of Dementia." *The Globe and Mail*, January 3. Available at: www.arch.mcgill.ca/prof/jemtrud/arch510/winter2009/neworleans/elisa%20costa/photos/Images%20for%20Presentation/http___license.icopyright.net_user_viewFreeUse.pdf. Last accessed February 15, 2013.

Plamper, Jan, and Benjamin Lazier. 2010. "Introduction: The Phobic Regimes of Modernity." *Representations* 110 (1): 58–65.

Raffel, Stanley. 1979. *Matters of Fact*. London, Boston, and Henley: Routledge & Kegan Paul.

Raffel, Stanley and Barry Sandywell, eds. 2016. *The Reflexive Initiative*. London: Routledge.

Schroeder, Steven, Marcus Krurpp, Lawrence Tierney, and Stephen McPhee. 1990. *Current Medical Diagnosis and Treatment*. Norwalk (CT): Appleton and Lange.

Schutz, Alfred. 1946. "The Well-Informed Citizen: An Essay on the Social Distribution of Knowledge." *Social Research* 13 (4): 463–78.

Simmel, Georg. (1918) 2010. *The View of Life: Four Metaphysical Essays with Journal Aphorisms*. Translated by John A.Y. Andrews and Donald N. Levine. Chicago: University of Chicago Press.

Žižek, Slavoj. 1997. *The Plague of Fantasies*. London: Verso.

9 Plague Strikes the Family

Introduction

Besides science and the novel, fact and fiction, the discourse on mortality that seems to materialize in the writing machine includes as part of its interpretive structure beliefs that are neither provable or testable but seem as if coherent figures of speech that seek to make facts meaningful and meanings factually relevant, various ways of transferring meaning we see as metaphoric and metonymic. For example, the sweep and currency of dementia as an apparent concerted tendency can be identified as a plague as if an impersonal force, perhaps without rhyme or reason and yet menacing and ever-present in the present. The notion of dementia as a plague is an interesting and provocative figure of speech that enables us to approach medical science as an order based upon notions of its legitimacy and validity that need to be opened to question if we are to engage ways in which the complexity of representations of dementia gloss their entanglement with anxiety over mortality.

The conception of dementia as an epidemic or, in an old-fashioned idiom, a plague, mechanizes the category as if it is corporeally driven much in the way of infection or infestation. Basically, the subject under such conditions can only react through plan and preparation to an unpredictable event, for the best intentions cannot overcome this contingency. Living under the sign of plague or of the infestation is living under the rule of the diabolical nihilist who can inflict a surprise anywhere and at any time. Such a subject, like Weber's Calvinist, can only orient methodically to rationalize everyday life in the areas deemed most vulnerable to the invasion. In its way everyday life becomes militarized, in the manner of a campaign waged by public health against the eruption of alterity reflected in the invasive intruder. Instead of an erotic or lovable relationship to Other expressed historically in much art, we are encouraged to accept the supervision of whatever technology the sciences of domestic management and planning have legitimized for administering everyday life. Thus, requirements of sanitation and nutrition, for example, are conceived as virtuous technologies for organizing the environment in terms of objectives of safety and security. Human vulnerability is typically reconfigured under the sign(s) of addiction and contagion in ways that require of leadership a pedagogy that is hypersensitive to the ambiguous mixture of force and nurturance in care. If the relationship between self-help and expertise frames the process of knowledge transmission, then the subject vulnerable to addiction must accept the authority of expertise without question in order to create a doctrine that can efficiently prepare for the emergency that is inevitable.

What I begin to suggest in this chapter is that if dementia is typically recognized as a plague due to a deteriorated faculty observable in great numbers of people, this attribution risks misrecognizing the plague as an affliction that is corporeal instead of seeing the possible source of danger to reside in the representation itself. In other words, the plague can make reference to the ways in which dementia is represented and so, could identify the infection as intellectual and of course linguistic, noting an externalization of thought that can appeal as intelligible to great numbers of people by simplifying the thought of dementia as if due to neurological factors rather than the paralyzing implications of imagining the destination of mortality in tune with the refrain of that "foreign intruder" in the mind.

Dementia, considered as an epidemic among the aged, attributable to brain dysfunctions, is increasingly recognized as a source of depression for the caregiver, causing negative experiences over the burdens of care, and leading to burnout. Though typically attributed to causes such as the severity of impairment, the difficulties of care, and the lack of adequate coping skills, it comes to be increasingly recognized that it is the perceived alienation of the dementia sufferer, his or her apparent distance and withdrawal, that might be the major cause of the caregiver's depression: Boss's research finds that the more a caregiver perceives a mate as psychologically absent the less masterful and the more depressed he or she is (Boss and Kaplan 1999). This sense of apathy and loss of motivation in the dementia sufferer seems a most powerful causal factor in the caregiver's experience, investing dementia with a degree of contagiousness where the subject appears to the caregiver as simultaneously physically present and psychologically absent, as an incarnation of abstraction and apartness. Why would the caregiver be depressed in the face of the confidence of the expert and the body of evidence to which expertise refers? To address this question we have to ask how expertise speaks about the plague and how it tries to prepare the vulnerable subject. In very many cases, public health claims that its expertise is disregarded or ignored by the subject and, because of this, policymaking tends to assume as its primary problem not simply the transfer of knowledge but the communication of its expertise as weighty and bona fide. Perhaps expertise runs up against the wall of language when its information is seen as missing the point.

This research conducted over the last thirty years in the field of family stress has found that stress introduced by diseases affects the ways in which individuals draw the boundaries of family membership, possibly causing confusion and dysfunction where the intimacy of the relationship to a loved one is qualified by the disease. This body of literature suggests that the subjective experience of family disintegration and reorganization is a decisive causal factor in producing depression and health problems for the caregiver (Boss *et al.* 1990; Boss and Kaplan 1999; Boss and Couden 2002). Looking specifically at dementia, these studies found that the disease stimulates uncertainty and ambiguity in the family because the patient is physically present but often psychologically absent, which raises disturbing questions about whether the person is "still there." Boss and Couden (2002) define "ambiguous loss" as the condition of not knowing whether a loved one is alive or dead, where a loved one is perceived as physically present while psychologically absent: "Our premise is that the most stressful losses are those that are ambiguous. When people are unable to obtain clarity about the status of a family member, they are often immobilized" (1352).

The model of family stress proposes a hypothetical causal sequence: the disease provokes boundary ambiguity, which contributes to caregiver confusion or disorientation, which leads to the need for clarification to work-through the loss. The importance of the family stress literature for our research is its suggestion of a powerful and demonstrable link of dementia to caregiver confusion/disorientation, which is revealed through quantification of how confusion (of roles, expectations, etc.) correlates with caregiver stress and depression (Boss and Couden 2002). Pauline Boss makes this point consistently through clinical cases from her practice that vividly exemplify this connection between ambiguity, confusion, and stress: "The frequently noted depression in caregivers may have more to do with the ambiguity of the loved one's absence or presence than with their heavy workload according to research" (Boss and Couden 2002, 1358–1359). In other words, this body of literature contends that when ambiguity is added to the caregiver's load, the task becomes even more difficult. In cases when the illness cannot be cured, "people must simultaneously hold two opposing ideas in their minds: the person as he or she was is gone; but the person is still here in my life" (1353).

If the depression of caregivers is connected to such conflicted conceptions of the sufferer as both present and absent, alive and dead, then we expect this lack of clarity to be a powerful factor in the caregiver's experience of the burdensome and depersonalized nature of the subjective experience. There is no evidence in support of the claim that more medical information or self-help advice can reduce such alienation and it cannot be expected to serve in such a way because self-help advice and even the most up-to-date medical and neurological information cannot give the caregiver anything more than an external sense of the situation, which still needs to be subjectively interpreted and clarified by the caregiver. That is, even if the caregiver is enabled to survive the situation more efficiently and to manage it more practically, we suspect that the depressing quality of the encounter must continue to haunt the relationship in ways that remain deleterious for those who provide care. It is this alienated figure of dementia that might result from an acute awareness of mortality and the limits of the life that seems to follow from what was named in another study (see Chapter 7; also Blum 2012) the Lear effect, after the story of King Lear and his ravings on the occasion of his abdication. This suggests that Lear's demented rant could be understood as part of his attempt to conceptualize the significance of his life and to elicit confirmation from intimates that his life mattered. We assume this question of mattering as fundamentally ambiguous and, when engaged as if a soliloquy, as a concern capable of inducing speech that risks appearing hallucinatory and incoherent. Thus the Lear effect is meant to describe the situation of dementia as a delusional translation of the question posed by a sufferer to and for oneself in ways that can only be observed by a caregiver as if hallucinatory and with depressing effects. The literature tends to confirm such an effect indirectly by identifying the caregiver's confusion in relation to the dementia sufferer as unsettling enough to be a cause of depression.

> Boss … conceptualized and found support for the theoretical premise that ambiguity regarding who is psychologically in and who is psychologically out of the family system can block family reorganization and accommodation to chronic stress… . Analyzing caregivers' perceptions of ambiguity in their family boundaries helps explain why some cope and some do not when faced with Alzheimer's disease. If the caregiver and family cannot perceptually clarify who is in and who is out of their family … the caregiver and family are immobilized.
>
> … The patient seems physically intact but, at the same time, is emotionally unavailable to the caregiver and other family members. Caregivers frequently say that their mates are no longer the person they used to know …
>
> (Boss *et al.* 1990, 2)

Being in the family is not self-evident, for one can be in and out at the same time. Such "inside" status might be closest to objective factors or the formal criterion as given by the category and the legitimate confirmation it assigns through the name, but all such classifications such as father, daughter, and the like, serve as beginnings or opportunities for imagining not only the rights, duties, and expectations that sociology identifies as statuses and roles, but the subjectivity of the incumbent, that problematic terrain that can always be treated as clear and unequivocal or, in contrast, as an unsettling open question. One hypothesis is that when the question is unsettling, other family members might experience such indefiniteness as a sign of dissatisfaction, and to be a consequence of the family (and its representatives) as not having done enough, of being responsible for the dissatisfaction. Thus, the perception of alienation as a signal of dissatisfaction can lower the self-regard of the others, say, of the caregiver, as if an effect that is contagious. So the plague can have a double effect, first on the vulnerable subject who becomes infected, and then on the intimate whose position as caregiver opens her or him to the contagious affliction.

Together and Apart

What are the conditions of boundary ambiguity, for being what Rancière calls together and apart at the same time? The connection of social change to the life cycle tells us that members of society have different relationships to participation in the society at different points of their life and that this can and does lead to differential involvement. This means that the enthusiasm that we identified after

Benjamin, for the present and its unprecedented character, is effected by the reversible influences of chronology that structure relations to time, to past and future, and to experiences of the contemporary (Blum, 2013). The most vivid example of such ambiguity resides in the spectacle of intergenerational division when the force of the present for the young often seems incomprehensible to those who are older. Agamben, after Nietzsche, formulates the relation to the contemporary in the best sense as being out of joint or untimely, or having the capacity to "see through" the present enthusiasm by "marking it above all as archaic" (2011, 10–19). Only those who perceive the indices and signatures of the archaic in the most modern and recent can be contemporary… . Both this distancing and nearness, which define contemporariness, have their foundation in this proximity to the origin that nowhere pulses with more force than in the present (Agamben 2011, 17). Enthusiasm is then not the *sine qua non* of the contemporary because "those who are truly contemporary, who truly belong to their time, are those who neither perfectly coincide with it nor adjust to its demands. They are thus in this sense irrelevant. But precisely because of this condition, precisely through this disconnection and anachronism, they are more capable than others of perceiving and grasping their own time. Contemporariness is, then, a singular relationship with one's own time, which adheres to it and at the same time, keeps a distance from it" (11). Here, while we risk inflating the alienation of boundary ambiguity as the poetic and reflective mode of Agamben's conception of the contemporary, we must recognize that his conception permits us to appreciate the apartness of boundary ambiguity as capable of reflectively engaging the enthusiasm of the present in ways that are not mechanical. It is this Grey Zone that boundary ambiguity begins to reveal in ways that can lead us to rethink the resonances of the contemporary that the supposed relation of aging and dementia can bring to mind.

War Story as Genre: Dementia Attacks the Family

On this note, we start with a human interest story in the Toronto press that recites the case of a vulnerable older person being attacked by the acronym FTD (frontotemporal dementia) that legitimates its externality, apparently affecting judgment and skill.

> Unlike Alzheimer's, which is more likely to strike older patients, FTD tends to hit people in their 40s, 50s and 60s, although patients can be diagnosed as early as their late 20s. Many people suffering from FTD are still caring for elderly parents, or, as in Mr. Shin's case, have young children.
>
> From 25 to 50 percent of FTD cases are believed to be hereditary, with the rest occurring sporadically in the population with no apparent genetic link. It is incurable.
>
> FTD attacks specific areas of the brain—the frontal and temporal lobes—causing nerve cells in those areas to shrink and die.

> The frontal lobe of the brain houses cells that affect a person's judgment, impulse control, social skills, and language abilities.
>
> As the cells in those areas atrophy and die, patients lose their ability to interact with others.
>
> They begin to act erratically, can develop compulsions, become indifferent to their families and withdraw from the world around them.
>
> In some cases, other areas of the brain are also affected, resulting in additional symptoms.
>
> (Hartley 2007: paragraphs 6–11)

The symptoms, erratic behavior, compulsion, and indifference are diagnosed by those who seem most familiar with him. What appears perplexing is the change and how to account for it in someone known because if it remains unexplained, the intimate bond itself can be put into question as if what is most secure, knowledge of the intimate, becomes Other. Just as the afflicted one is seen to be "attacked" in his brain, so is the family member "attacked" by this eruption. The first question the story considers is how this attack takes shape in the person designated, appearing it seems as if a sign of his depression that puzzles and comes to depress his intimates. The first question posed asks how we are to understand his changed behavior.

Being Emotionally Flat = More Than Depression

> Three years ago, Mr. Shin lost his job as the manager of a dress-manufacturing company. The company said it was a result of cost-cutting layoffs, but, thinking back, his wife isn't so sure. Mr. Shin had worked there for more than 20 years and his late father had been a pillar of the company for more than 30. She now believes her husband was let go because of the early symptoms of his condition. It was the first sign that something was wrong.
>
> "About six months after he lost his job, he didn't seem to be motivated in trying to determine what his next steps were going to be," she says. "Because his dad had died the year before and then he lost his job, I thought it was depression."
>
> Mrs. Shin tried to give her husband space, despite his growing moodiness and apathy, but he didn't initiate conversation with her any more [sic] and when they did speak, they argued. He would scream at the kids over things that never upset him before.
>
> He signed up for a real-estate-training course, twice, but dropped out. A bartending course brought the same result. Money got tight, and Mr. Shin

didn't seem to care. Soon, the couple were sleeping in different beds and on the verge of divorce.

> "He was emotionally flat," she recalls. "He was unable to see anything beyond himself and became very focused on just his little world. I just couldn't understand why Michael was like this."
>
> (Hartley 2007: paragraphs 13–17)

Explanations introduced include factors such as his loss of a job, which seemed to create a lack of motivation and disinterest in the present. Because his father died, a connection is made to depression as if the death of his father "made" him depressed as a mechanical contagious exchange. Yet here, space is created for rethinking the causal impact of his father's death as something other than a simple empirical exchange, but as a provocation stimulating him to engage the meaning of life and death that a father's death might reveal. This range of factors such as loss of job, rejection, father's death, are cited while yet ignored as rich conditions or "thick" meanings, simply to be treated as background for introducing the brain as a causal agent. But there is no reason for deferring the need to work-through the situation and the appearance of the father as a meaningful social phenomenon, showing the brain's use possibly as a premature rush to resolve an apparently ambiguous situation occasioned by the enigma of the father's subjectivity. His wife can only see him as "emotionally flat" and now in hindsight can reconstruct his dismissal from his job a reasonable response of the employer to signs of premature brain damage rather than as the cost-cutting maneuver she had been led to believe. As an illustration of Garfinkel's (1967) use of the documentary method, she finds that all along he had been damaged goods. Thus, apparently unequipped to engage what is happening except as infractions of expectations, she searches for an account that might situate the changes. Here, we can suggest an alternative: stimulated by his father's death to think about mortality and irretrievable loss, he reflects upon what *he* will lose in death and what there is in his life worth holding onto. What could it all matter to a wide-awake person, factors such as ambition, future, real-estate jobs, bartending, even his wife and the children?

Signs of Withdrawal

> As the months went by, the family's situation grew more dire. Mr. Shin had no concept of time, began taking his kids to the wrong hockey rinks for games and even though he was eating junk food all the time—something he never did before—he was still losing weight. He looked weak. He started to shake. His spine started to curve. He didn't walk so much as stumble around the house.
>
> Mr. Shin feared he might be developing Lou Gehrig's disease (amyotrophic lateral sclerosis or ALS), which had killed his father.

> Mrs. Shin nearly had to drag her husband to see the family doctor, who recommended that he see a therapist. But after a few sessions, it became clear the problem wasn't psychological. It was something much worse.
>
> (Hartley 2007: paragraphs 18–20)

We have to begin to engage the structure of indifference because the lack of concentration so apparent in this history of infractions can just as well be reflected upon as a kind of self-absorption, an intense concentration that fuels the infelicities. How can it be said here that it became "clear" that the problem was something "worse" than psychological and what kind of advice is honored in this talk? Presumably as a causal force, the brain is "worse" because it is unalterable, but such a self-congratulatory gesture on the part of a science tends to assume somehow that what is "worse" now because biological can only become "better" with the progress and march of medical science. Yet, what is truly "worse" in this exchange might be the condition of death itself, which this science can never alter. It is clear though that everyone is on the same page here, countering Dad's fantasies with expert consultation.

> Mr. Shin had always been an excellent driver, but in February of 2006 he started getting into strange car accidents. In one frightening incident, he reversed into a car on Highway 7 in Markham after missing the driveway he was looking for. That July, he hit a parked car on the street outside his house. He told his wife that it was a small accident, but in reality the family van was totaled. The police were called and Mr. Shin was nearly charged with dangerous driving.
>
> The accidents alone cost the family more than $10,000 and Mr. Shin, who always had been organized about money, seemed to have lost all concept of finances.
>
> He was talked into spending $8,000 on personal training, nutritional counseling and a personal trainer at a local gym.
>
> Three different companies were fertilizing the family's lawn at one point because they would cold-call the house and Mr. Shin would agree to have them come by. After a salesman came to the door one day, he switched the family's Internet and phone service to a new company at a higher price.
>
> It wasn't long before Mrs. Shin had to start pulling money out of the family's RRSPs to cover basic costs. Now, she's not sure how she's going to be able to afford to send her kids to university.
>
> "He would make Internet purchases until bill paying became an issue, because it wasn't even happening," she says. "He'd just spend and then he didn't ever pay anything so the notices would come and we were in danger of having the credit card cut off."

> Mr. Shin started developing uncontrollable eating habits. He would use half the bottle of salad dressing at a single meal. He nearly caused a fire when he left a bag of popcorn in the microwave for more than 10 minutes. He became incontinent, stopped bathing, and once soiled himself at a family picnic. The kids stopped bringing their friends around. Mrs. Shin wondered how much more she could take.
>
> (Hartley 2007: paragraphs 21–27)

Signs of Decline

Perhaps mortality puts into relief the pathos of this family. Accidents are one thing and can be a result of lack of concentration, stemming from the aforementioned indifference and distraction, but financial problems are not amusing either to society or to families of loved ones. Eating habits, carelessness, and incontinence are disturbing signs open to the family but in ways always shadowed by the possibility that Mr. Shin could not care less. The force of withdrawal and disengagement needs to be explored before imagining more reassuring accounts.

> In December of 2006, Mr. Shin was finally diagnosed with FTD by doctors at Sunnybrook Hospital in Toronto.
>
> Mrs. Shin feels like she has lost almost everything. She started dating her husband when she was just 16, when they met at an event at a Japanese cultural center 33 years ago, and the pair have been together ever since.
>
> "We never talked a lot about the future," she says. "I just figured we'd continue the way we were. We were very comfortable in the relationship that we had."
>
> …
>
> When the diagnosis came, "I knew already," Mrs. Shin says. "I had read everything I could get my hands on already… . I said I needed to know what kind of variant it was. I said I was prepared. But you're not really prepared.
>
> "There was almost a sense of relief, knowing that somebody is actually telling me now as opposed to me trying to guess what it was. Because this is such an uncommon disease, trying to figure out exactly what it was, was pretty stressful," she says.
>
> (Hartley 2007: paragraphs 28–30, 34–35)

What is it that a wife would want in order to relieve this anxiety? Not to be blamed or held responsible and above all to be reassured that nothing has really changed, that the change, when conceived as external, is no one's fault, something beyond our control. The spouse here needs to hold on to the dream and though crushed by the disappointing loss, feels fortified by the "hard" explanation. It is worth considering how the wife's investment in the situation (the intimacy, the dream) is frustrated by the "new" indifference and change in the person, motivating her to qualify what she had assumed and expected of herself and the other alone and together. It is important for this wife to understand herself as a victim of external conditions rather than as a collaborator in a relationship that is fine-tuning itself to an awareness of mortality. What his wife does not want to honor and what we should see clearly is her inability to share with Mr. Shin and his experience, to achieve the intimacy necessary for witnessing his ordeal rather than externalizing it. Right now, we rely upon the brain to do this work.

Expertise

We can only groan at the doctor despite the gravity of a situation like this, finding it difficult to elevate her view to encompass anything other than the brain despite the social character of these infractions.

> Sandra Black, who officially diagnosed Mr. Shin, has been treating FTD patients for close to a decade and has seen the devastating results.
>
> "It's an extremely difficult disease on the families," says Dr. Black, who is the head of neurology at Sunnybrook Health Sciences Centre in Toronto.
>
> "I think it's just about the worst imaginable, because the person starts to lose their sense of others and the needs of others. So for a spouse, you lose the person in a whole different way."
>
> …
>
> Like Alzheimer's, an FTD diagnosis is a death sentence. Although some patients live as long as eight years after the symptoms first occur, most don't make it that far. "Sadly there are [no treatments]," Dr. Black says. "There are some things that we're trying out. It's so much rarer than Alzheimer's, so it hasn't had the same attention."
>
> Alzheimer's patients retain many of their social skills for some time after symptoms begin. They can be affectionate, even clingy, but family members generally don't initially get the feeling that they are unwanted or unappreciated.
>
> As Mr. Shin became more withdrawn and detached, Mrs. Shin had to explain to her children that their father didn't mean to laugh when they fell down, but just didn't know how to react any more.
>
> "With frontotemporal dementia, you get someone who no longer gives a damn about you or anyone else. They no longer feel. They no longer care,"

> Dr. Black says. "They're not happy when a child graduates or something good happens. They don't feel bad when a mother dies. It's really hard and usually it has a big effect on the marital relationship."
>
> She says FTD often causes people to do things they never would have done before. They have lost the ability to see themselves through the eyes of others, so they don't understand why people are shocked or appalled.
>
> "I remember one case of a grandfather, a very respectable man, who started molesting children in his neighborhood," Dr. Black says. "He actually got arrested and we had to do everything we could to prevent him from going to jail."
>
> One of the first patients Dr. Black ever diagnosed with FTD was a school principal who began to behave in ways that were upsetting his family. They suspected something was amiss with him, but couldn't put their finger on it.
>
> During a dinner party one night, the principal got up from his chair, walked to the corner of the dining room and urinated on the floor. He was diagnosed with FTD a short time later.
>
> "I remember my patients with this condition very vividly, because each person is so unique and the suffering that went on somehow strikes you because there aren't that many," Dr. Black says.
>
> "I've learned about and lived through these diseases with patients in a way that gives you a lot of respect for how it can destroy lives, often young lives."
>
> (Hartley 2007: paragraphs 31–33, 36–45)

In attributing such signs immediately to reassuring FTD, the doctor forecloses thinking through the situation as such and how it might contribute socially to depersonalization as not caring, not feeling, and not being able to take the perspective of others. This formulaic identification of psychopathic behavior needs more than the hasty and ungrounded rush to a genetic formulation. If this is the authoritative way of addressing psychopathic behavior, then how can we place the Nuremburg trials of Nazis and indeed, our enmity to all those we have treated as villains or sought to destroy? Here, what seems uncanny is the change in conduct of an apparently "normal" person as if suddenly perverse, doing malicious or unsociable behavior that would have been unthinkable in the past.

Lacking an experimental design to control for all extraneous variables to try to assess the cause of the change, such treatment avoids looking at the situation of the afflicted as a particular kind of relationship at this point in life. Here, the list of horror cases of FTD appears in the format of a canon adjudicated by expertise that has seen many kinds, all examples of upright and normal figures turning overnight into ghouls much like the benign serial killer next door, or the unassuming terrorist.

First, there is an absence of affect (reminiscent of Meursault in Camus' *Étranger* who showed no remorse, asking if he might smoke at his mother's funeral), then the grandfather turned molester (inviting us to question whether Roman Polanski had shrinking brain cells or amyloid plaque), to the school principal urinating at the dinner party (and what might he have been trying to say at that gathering?). This unreflective litany can only cause us to consider how such appeals to the brain might begin to create possibilities for legal defenses as alternatives to not-guilty-by-reason-of-insanity pleas as if the format could legitimate exoneration in ways that give everyone relief. Here, it is worth asking what such molecular idealism does to the place of truth, falsity, and accountability (and perhaps, as Baudrillard suggests, we might need to disclose the purgation of meaning as its true value).

Indifference as an Impasse

Is the indifference noted of the sufferer personal or impersonal? And even more, if everyone is suffering, who is suffering from what in this situation? This strange question asks us to consider if the absence of affect disclosed by the father shows its own affectivity as a shape of contempt for the family and its round of life, or if not, how it reflects a condition outside of everyone's control that can be treated as a sign not of wrath or negativity but as a reflection of the workings of the world and life as a natural process. Granted that the impersonality of the father's indifference might be felt sorrowfully or as painful, it is still not to be read as an accusation directed personally against the family and its life. In fact, despite the horror of the condition and its inscrutability, it might be a relief to know that such indifference is unmotivated, a result of conditions over which we have no control.

There is no room for accusation and assignments of personal responsibility here because the attribution of causal force to the brain can deny agency to the others, whether the mother and the family environment or the father himself. The impasse created by the spectacle of such indifference makes it possible to withdraw judgment, absolving all from blame for the changed situation. Now we can safely say that the Ought is dead and the inevitable ambiguity it is capable of releasing has expired because nobody in this situation can be held responsible, not simply for what befalls the father, but for thinking about what has happened here. In other words, the elimination of judgment is an elimination of thought, of thinking about what the father is orienting to, since he like everyone else is seen simply as a victim of impersonal conditions inherent in the deterioration of corporeal faculties.

The plague we suffer from then is not inflicted by dementia and its inevitable appearance as a correlative condition of aging but in the myth as punishment by the Gods for the collective acceptance of simplistic explanation, punishing us for our will to relinquish the desire to think about the deterioration of the subject by reflecting upon its possible meaning, choosing instead to substitute for such desire an easy acceptance of clear and convenient neurological speculation. We are afflicted by the force of neurology itself as an intellectual formula, the format of molecular idealism that can silence our desire to take up the phenomenon as a matter for reflection. Could the indifference of the father be created not by dementia but by the indifference he assumes of the others who he sees as treating his aging as demented rather than as reflectively attuned to mortality? Mimetic contagion suggests that his indifference to them might mirror their indifference to the mortal implications of his passage. Is there a way in which his indifference to (their) life and their indifference to (his) death be reconciled not in a reparative synthesis but in mutually oriented action of some form? In the idiom of Alfred Schutz, can they learn jointly to make music together? This gives us a glimpse of the impasse.

Line of Descent

> Mr. Shin's brother, Stephen, lives in Florida and usually comes north to Toronto to visit his family several times a year. However, in the past 36 months, with each passing visit, he was shocked at the rapid decline in his brother's health.
>
> "He's a different person, it's like he took an aging pill," Stephen says. "I see he's so different than he was before. I think that's really what strikes me. I find myself overcompensating when we talk. You look at this shell, and you wonder if maybe there just isn't anything going on up there. It's just not the way it should be."
>
> When he looks at his gaunt, unsteady, and confused brother, Stephen remembers the devoted father and husband who "did laundry like it was the army" and drove the kids everywhere.
>
> "I was so impressed with the way they worked as a team, as a marriage," he says. "Because June had to get up early, Michael used to get the kids up, feed them, and he'd have all their books and their bags lined up at the front door with the shoes they were going to wear beside their jackets."
>
> Because Michael suffers from FTD and his father died of ALS, Stephen has started to worry about his own health. "I look at Michael now, and I hate to say this, but I think, 'Oh my gosh, I really need to go and see if it is genetic,'" he says. "It scares me. It scares me a great deal."
>
> (Hartley 2007: paragraphs 54–58)

The new narrative of extinction, reiterating the destruction of a line or of a people, passing though pogrom, genocide, holocaust, and collective violence of such atrocious magnitude, can now be imagined as the vengeance of the body and the line of genetics, capable of making collectives disappear in the absence of accountability, fostering a passivity and hopelessness that even diet and exercise will not be able to cure. Perhaps the hope here is that the research of medicine will, with sufficient funding, reach the point where even such death can be mastered.

Now we can appreciate the two-sided nature of the plague as a collective representation: on the one hand, its horrific character can infect and destroy populations, while on the other hand, by virtue of the impersonality of its corporeal source, it can seem to exempt all from responsibility. The plague can eliminate agency or the most vital part of oneself by standardizing its effects as if results of a destruction almost generic, and so, totally unlike a holocaust, genocide, or diaspora, but with similar overtones. Note how the plague functions like the market as a symbol of impersonal growth and decline beyond anyone's control, a sign of the impotence of human agency. The plague, beyond good and evil, reveals that no one is responsible for it, and yet, one can be determined as culpable in not being an adequate and committed consumer of the information transmitted by the science of planning and engineering. Responsibility belongs to those who turn away from the expertise of public health (or in the case of the market, from investment planning, or from doctrines of social engineering), those who turn away from the advice to accept the best practices of self-help and self-care. It is not the machine that is seen as responsible and its systemic policies and counsel to work, to be productive, to live and love in the present and to accept life and its imperfections as it is here and now, but this subject whose resistance seems to show careless and antisocial indifference in the figure of non-compliance. Responsibility is attributed to the imperfection of knowledge transfer and the mechanics of the machine, which might be rectified by rehabilitation that pays attention to knowledge dissemination as technology. Communication, shifted to the center and redefined, is now reactivated in terms of the postal model of transfer as another gesture in the age-old colonization of the vulnerable psyche. If life inflicts upon its subject the experience of loss, then the risk of life is that it can be viewed as an affliction.

Dementia as Sacrificial Violence: Meaning as Culprit

In René Girard's work, the myth of the plague ([1972] 1977) represents it as inflicted upon a community as if punishment by the Gods (or unnamed forces) for a crime it is suspected of having committed for expelling the force of the sacred from its life (and city) and typically, for a gesture that tends to reveal a reverence for the profane as necessary for the survival of the city. The sacred is viewed as a superstitious distraction diverting the community from reality and is expelled on these utilitarian grounds as if it interferes with the perpetuity of the city. Note that the sacred makes reference in the primordial sense not to theology, superstition, or even the "magic" that we have come to identify it with, but to the fundamental ambiguity intrinsic to the notion of meaning and value. In this sense, what is seen as the crime against the sacred is the renunciation of any commitment to the Ought or to the value-laden character of all words and deeds. In other words, the community is punished for its systemic indifference to any concern for value and meaning, imposing in this way a stain upon it for its single-minded mechanical solidarity, its automated attempt at unanimity achieved at the expense of a more organic solidarity (see Durkheim [1893] 1933). In this sense, the unhappiness, stress, and frustration of a modern community such as ours might be understood as an infliction of the plague upon us as punishment for our indifference to meaning that is disclosed in our collective fixation upon the externalization of language and, in this case, the rush to neurological explanations for what can only remain enigmatic.

The hypothesis (story) of what this community imagines sees it as doing what it does to honor practical and utilitarian ends in order to achieve the communal prosperity that it thinks requires it to exclude an attentiveness to the sacred in order to make a place for efficient, practical action because contemplation of the enigma released by the force of the sacred in life produces conundrums of meaning that lead to indecision, anxieties, irreconcilable disputes and subjective caprice; yet attaining unity in such a way can also result in a simplified and superficial focus upon life devoid of spirit or substance. To expel the sacred might be akin to creating a bargain with the devil on the grounds that it makes life easier to bear. But the intermittent and precocious intuition of mortality as our common fate always shows that the devil returns to extract his due in the absence of the sacred as the fundamental anxiety that underlies all affective perturbation. Before considering how the fixation upon neurological accounts fits this formula, it will be worthwhile returning to the story of Oedipus as the primordial Greek story of the plague and the retribution it suggests because Greek tragedy illustrates in picturesque ways how the loss of the sacred infects life by dramatizing the way dependency upon the Ought is a necessity of life that the city risks obscuring.

If as the story goes, Prometheus gave us the means of repressing the thought of death in order to embrace our present, Benardete is right to say: "The condition for the possibility of tragedy is post-Promethean, for what it presents is pre-Promethean man, for whom death is before his eyes and there is neither art nor hope. In taking us outside ourselves, tragedy makes us experience our total dependence on gods. The abyss over which they suspend us reveals our need of them (Benardete 2000, 108).

The sickness of the collective as a spiritual entity is parodied in the story of the plague that resurrects it as if a corporeal body vulnerable to a disease by which it is attacked. This is to say that a community that renounces the sacred is like a corporeal body divested of spirit. In the absence of a commitment to a conception of dialogue that can bind the collective even in its differences, the body can only explode in a series of convulsive actions and reactions that display sensitivity in a circuit of acrimonious exchanges. The primary symptom of this sick society is its pattern of acting out disclosed in the disagreements by which it is seen to be animated in its exchanges of opinions that resemble an adversarial struggle. Girard calls the violence mimetic and contagious because everyone imitates the aggression of the other as if fear for one's being is at stake and one's gain is the other's loss and vice versa in a zero-sum interaction. Such a cycle is modeled after an Oedipal dialectic in which one aspires to possess what is lacked (interpretive finality) and fears losing what is possessed (interpretive finality). Violence is only arrested by bonding together in uniformity against a victim who is made to stand for the extinction of the sacred. Girard's notion of the king as scapegoat shows how the leader can be made to stand for the failure of resolve of the community itself, as a surrogate criminal that represents the criminality of the community.

This format fits the picture of a collective defending itself from recognizing the implications of the irresolute Grey Zone through its construction of a formula that defers resentment much in the way the perplexity of the relation of body to mind is pacified by identifying the mind and its propensity towards mediation as the reason for the plague, making the affective excess of thought responsible for the discord. The plague makes tacit reference to the view of dialogue as gratuitous talk animated by a concerted affective investment that prevents the community from achieving real results, i.e. acting in concert. More than mind, the complexity of meaning is sacrificed by biomedicine to achieve a resolution that is simple and capable of engendering unanimity. This of course is an age-old tactic of science and the mimetic violence it perpetuates on affect and its "subjectivity." Moreover, this serves Girard's purpose for using the conception as a paradigm of collective acting-out that seems to him to characterize any society remaining unreflective in relation to the ambiguity of its normative order and the authority it sanctifies by masking it in an appeal to a simple unifying format. In this way the collective defers recognizing the conventionality of its order. This is the standard Weberian model of the normative order, buttressed by his conceptions of legitimacy and validity (the legitimate order, the valid order) that both anchors social life and opens it to challenge. Girard identifies this challenge as a sacrificial crisis that collective life harbors at its core as an essential incommensurability (see Rancière [1995] 1999 on this incommensurability) and that marks its symbolic order as constantly and productively contentious.

Following René Girard, what if we treat the story of biomedicine as the evolution of a myth? The identification of the scapegoat displaces recognition of the limits of the collective. Let us propose that the collective must be insecure about the relation of body to mind not as a sign of its deficiency but for the reason of the fundamental enigma of this relationship. If the story leads to identifying the affectivity of mind as culprit for the plague (as the seat of affective distortion), then this is because this insecurity of the collective has been and continues as a source of rancorous conflict unless arrested by a formula that can unify and provide resolution.

The formula compels the following story. As a source of overstimulation that draws people away from the truth, affective distortion is viewed as causing the error of an ignorance of science in a way that targets it as a scapegoat for the fact of collective perplexity and as a catalyst of the conflict of opinions. The model of knowledge transfer argues that people will receive the truth when their affect can be managed in ways that release them from the self-interest and self-indulgence that causes intransigent relations to the speech of expertise. Irony towards the claims of expertise, even if ungrounded, is considered antisocial, a resistance fuelled by excessive self-affectation. Violence is directed against meaning by inflicting upon all speakers a model of exposition that imitates the simple postal transmission of information and by expelling any figurativeness that cannot be economized in clichés that command immediate recognition (in literature, Jennifer Ashton [2003] has discussed this violence in many shapes).

The use of the brain defers resentment by unifying all against meaning (unless neurologically or chemically diagnosed and described simplistically), whether as a source of disease or a normal causal sequence. Connotations of mindedness evoked by the brain as a seat of thought are reformulated by purging any desire for a reflective engagement with conceptions, methods of confirmation, and graphic models of patterning and interconnection that display it as anything other than an elegant bit of machinery modeled after the solar system, describable as such and nothing more. The primordial sense of wonder that is often taken to inaugurate philosophy at its origin is redefined to simulate the breathless exclamations of roller-coaster passengers, or spectators in the planetarium who seem reverentially transfixed by its sublime mock-up of the universe, or urban tourists held in thrall by architectural spectacle. The brain is redesigned as a figure from its seat as the core of the voluptuous unruliness of mind into its spectacle as an elegant bit of machinery that makes the collective spellbound. Still, the real guilty party is not the brain (nor the mind) but the imagined relationship to its insecurity that is viewed as preventing the collective from developing a discriminating commitment to reflection. Mind itself is not expelled because its status as complex can be easily reduced to the image of a cognitive system modeled after a network of corporeal exchanges written up as a complicated system of variables. Similarly, affectivity can be simulated as a circuit of neural transactions in such a mock-up of thought. Since the collective, reduced to a horde, always appears to be infected by contentiousness in adversarial exchanges of opinion that only seem to lead to irresolution, uniformity in agreements that are achieved consensually and step-wise without dialogue (or without "talky-talk" as a colleague of mine once called it), is always appealed to as the final resting place for quieting conflicting opinion. The use of the brain in biomedical formulae can defer temptations to escalate resistance to such simplified talk.

In this current chapter, the Chin family suffers for the society and its insecurity, sacrificing an engagement with dementia as a meaningful and inconclusive encounter by assigning responsibility to the deterioration of faculties as culprit because they are told by experts how research confirms that the brain is the seat of dementia. The real culprit however is the desire to think otherwise, which the wife treats now as a temptation she has happily overcome. It is not the wife's fault, for she is a victim used by the society to displace its ignorance about dementia. An even more dramatic choice of victim would be the sufferer whose thoughts about mortality are construed as hallucinatory in the absence of any evidence. The horde simply does not know what it is talking about and chooses the family to displace its insecurity. Doctors of medicine stand in as pundits in such a chain of significations. Yet the doctor, too, is a victim of this lack of knowledge about dementia and its causes that have to be filled in by opinions that can resolve the perplexity. The doctor operates on hearsay no different than the wife. That affectivity is now the culprit simply reverses the age-old priority of the use of the brain as scapegoat in those schools of philosophy that once viewed it as a seat of distortion or irrelevance. Whether mind or body, what we see is that these elections serve as figures for masking the insecurity of the collective and the need to build mythology in order to arrest interminable sacrificial conflict. Yet, this insecurity cannot be resolved by another doctrine or opinion that simply extends the debate by incorporating every intended resolution as another voice in the circuit of actions. The virtue of death is not that it reveals again such ungroundedness but that it dramatizes the need for meaningful action to be taken under such conditions. This need for action in the face of an impasse has been formulated, especially by Arendt, as judgment or for the decision here-and-now in the absence of any conclusive support or as Socrates says, of a ground plan for the action "down to the last detail." This need for judgment in relation to the Ought is what qualifies the fantasy of inexorability that rules the algorithm and discloses its reductionism as both reassuring and simpleminded.

The implication of the figure of plague is that if we assume in retaliation that biomedicine is the culprit, we risk reciprocating such violence by making its position into a scapegoat. The interminable exchanges of acting out between reciprocally wronged and victimized speakers can only be overcome by assuming a position that enables us to appreciate the "real" culprit as the collective itself and its normative order, not as malign but as a necessarily imperfect (complex) system. Note that the same order can and has honored both extremes of body and mind as bases for unity and has and can expel both body and mind respectively as victims. Such a normative order can fluctuate in its evaluations because its decisions are not only ungrounded but unreflected and untheorized. Note that though a solution is impossible, reflection and theorizing is not and has to continue in relation to such impossibility and to such incapacity. This further fits Rancière's formula that views the absence of politics as the absence of such a space for concerted reflection. Thus, the sacrificial crisis identifies the collective not as ungrounded, which is inevitable, but more pertinently as unreflective in relation to its ungroundedness. Yet despite what we might assert about the deficiency and arbitrary norms, the normative order cannot be a culprit since it simply must disclose the "hole" in Being upon which it is based, the unreason at the heart of its apparatus. This incommensurability or contingency (whatever we call it) is the basis for the action that might make its limits transparent.

In terms of dementia, biomedicine does not make mind the culprit, because it tries to colonize mind as that organ that needs to be objectified in order to be an object for reproducible discourse. The culprit for biomedicine is neither mind nor affect but soft-hearted and unscientific conceptions of research that are not up-to-date in any present concerning the advances of science. Whether neurology or genetics, affect is redefined in any way legitimated by lay appeals to results of "research" in order to make its representation enforceably intelligible for a collection of common speakers. As the ambiguity that is expelled, the scapegoat can be personified in any action seen as ruled by the desire for mediation (and meditation), by any concern for meaning (see Arendt 1978 on the difference between truth and meaning). We see the real victim as the minded and subjective relationship to dementia or to anything (and its corporeal symptoms) reflected in the sufferer or intimates, and caregiver(s). Thus, the plague of dementia is perpetrated on a community for disengaging from any encounter with its meaning, for surrendering to the easy acceptance of the stipulation of the body as its cause. We are all victims, dementia sufferer, family, caregiver, doctors, medical science, and you and I. The ease in accepting the stipulation discloses by analogy its correlation to an acceptance of the scapegoat as the stipulation of a mob, tyrant, or of any figure alerting us to a very complex system of accusation and reduction in politics and in language, revealing how the figure of the plague operates in the mob rule of politics, life, and language most often as the necessity in majority rule. In contrast to such convenience, it is instructive to appreciate that this contentious exchange, inevitable in a diverse society, is precisely the scene of the "argumentative plot" that Rancière ([1992] 1995, 102, 104, 105, 106) identifies as the normal modus operandi of democracy.

> Imparity is an essential part of democracy… . The only kind of dialogue compatible with democracy is one where the parties hear one another but do not agree with one another… . Grievance is the true measure of otherness, the thing that unites interlocutors while simultaneously keeping them at a distance from each other… . Depoliticizing conflicts in order to settle them, or stripping otherness of any yardstick the better to solve its problem—this is the madness which our time identifies with a reasonable and easy democracy.

It might be that accusation and victimization of self and other is part of this imparity that reveals dialogue under such conditions as sufficiently hyperbolic to produce a vitality that is two-sided, energizing, and accusatory, part of what Lacan identifies as hysterical.

> But difference does not mean the assumption of the different identity or the plain confrontation of two identities. The place for the working out of difference is … the *topos* of an argument. And the place for such an argument is an interval … or a gap; being together to the extent that we are in-between.
>
> (Rancière 1992, 62)

In other words, irresolute difference is the foundation of dialogue that can only display the disagreement itself as the locus of the dialogue, meaning that the "real object" of any dialogue is the Grey Zone as it is disclosed in the disagreements elicited by a specific content or commonplace in relation to the alternative paths of action it motivates:

> Disagreement is not the conflict between one who says white and another who says black. It is the conflict between one who says white and another who also says white but does not understand the same thing by it or does not understand that the other is saying the same thing in the name of whiteness… . Disagreement occurs wherever contention over what speaking means constitutes the very rationality of the speaking situation… . It is the choice of the very measuring rod.
>
> (Rancière [1995] 1999, x, xx, 5)

This suggests that the end of dialogue is the agreement it envisions in making the "choice of the very measuring rod" its focus.

> The foundation of politics … is the lack of foundation, the sheer contingency of any social order… . It is … the incommensurable at the heart of the distribution of speaking bodies.
>
> (Rancière [1995] 1999, 16, 19)

Conclusion

Girard's image of sacrificial crisis and the plague it narrates, when divested of its theological implications, can be a resource for politics, that is, for a dialogical conception of the political, when we can overcome the propensity towards reciprocal violence and acting out that follow from the oppositional impulses of our togetherness and apartness in relation to the collective, by seeing ourselves as *both* Same and Other. The hysterical affect released in the sacrificial crisis can result in both the tenacity to defend oneself against objectification, and to strive to maintain oneself as more than we can say, in ways liberating at its best and self-indulgent at its worst. According to Anspach (2004, xxxiii), by converting Nietzsche's maxim "the edge of wisdom is turned against the wise man" into "the twist of the wise man is the one who turns the edge of wisdom against himself," Girard discloses the truth of the identity of oneself with the others and, we might add, empowers his difference by virtue of this recognition. This is a reinstatement of Hegel's formula for the *aufheben* that counsels us to cancel the opposition and to preserve the difference (Birchall 1981). Such an ambiguous position can lead us to ask if the search for self-knowledge is yet another such facile cliché and, if so, whether the nihilist might be correct. Thus, if the value of death is not simply its ontological status, it can be seen to be functional in its curious way by causing us to reflect upon conditions that could revitalize a present. In this space resides the ambiguity we call a Grey Zone, causing us to ponder not whether death is good or bad, but how it exists as a condition that we must engage in one way or another to make it eventful, to use it as real equipment for living.

References

Agamben, Giorgio. 2011. *Nudities*. Stanford, CA: Stanford University Press.
Anspach, Mark R. 2004. "Editor's Introduction: Imitating Oedipus." In *Oedipus Unbound: Selected Writings on Rivalry and Desire* by René Girard, edited by Mark A. Anspach, vii–liv. Stanford: Stanford University Press.
Benardete, Seth. 2000. "On Plato's 'Phaedo.'" In *The Argument of the Action: Essays on Greek Poetry and Philosophy*, 277–296. Chicago: University of Chicago Press.
Birchall, B.C. 1981. "Hegel's Notion of *Aufheben*." *Inquiry* 24 (1): 75–103.
Blum, Alan. 2012. "The Enigma of the Brain and its Place as Cause, Character, and Pretext in the Imaginary of Dementia." *History of the Human Sciences* 25 (4): 108–124.
___. 2013. "Aging as a Social Form: The Phenomenology of the Passage." *Journal of Medical Humanities* 35: 19–36.

Boss, Pauline, Wayne Caron, Joan Horbal, and James Mortimer. 1990. "Prediction of Depression in Caregivers of Dementia Patients: Boundary Ambiguity and Mastery." *Family Process* 29 (3): 245–254. (Chp. 9).

Boss, Pauline and Lori Kaplan. 1999. "Depressive Symptoms among Spousal Caregivers of Institutionalized Mates with Alzheimer's: Boundary Ambiguity and Mastery as Predictors." *Family Process* 38 (1): 85–103. (Chp. 9).

Boss, Pauline and Barbara A. Couden. 2002. "Ambiguous Loss from Chronic Physical Illness: Clinical Interventions with Individuals, Couples, and Families." *Psychotherapy in Practice* 58 (11): 1351–1360. (Chp. 9).

Durkheim, Émile. (1893) 1933. *The Division of Labor in Society*. Translated by George Simpson. New York: The Free Press.

Garfinkel, Harold. 1967. *Studies in Ethnomethodology*. Englewood Cliffs, NJ: Prentice Hall.

Girard, René. (1972) 1977. *Violence and the Sacred*. Translated by Patrick Gregory. Baltimore: The Johns Hopkins University Press.

Hartley, Matt. 2007. "A Disappearing Dad." *The Globe and Mail*, November 17. Available at www.theglobeandmail.com/incoming/a-disappearing-dad/article698128/?page=all. Last accessed May 1, 2014.

Rancière, Jacques. (1992) 1995. "Politics, Identification, Subjectivization." *October* 61: 58–64.

——. (1995) 1999. *Disagreement: Politics and Philosophy*. Translated by Julie Rose. Minneapolis: University of Minnesota Press.

10 The Cliché of Depression

Introduction

We might risk making biomedicine, its materialist sources and nihilistic overtones, a scapegoat for the intermittent sense of life being askew. Yet Wittgenstein's counsel that we should not tell someone they are in error, but show them the road from error to truth, is important to remember. What are we to do with affect, with longing and resignation that Simmel identifies as our primary affects, or how should we live life in the shadow of death: forget it, deny it, or repress it?

Depression and burnout of the caregiver for a dementia sufferer is reputed to have reached epic proportions in North America and Europe and typically more neurological information and self-help advice is recommended as antidotes for relieving caregiver distress (Blum 2016). I have suggested that the depression of the caregiver is not simply a function of helplessness with respect to the physical conditions but is connected to an inability to express what needs expressing, some kind of response to the situation of dementia that is more than palliative.

I propose that for the caregiver to understand the dementia sufferer it seems necessary to orient to the inarticulate experience of the death of anyone, including oneself, the caregiver, and the unspoken and obscene sense of "futureless future" (Lingis 2000) that death expresses. The otherness within is a figure of speech for our unconscious, the ambiguous and unsettling fear of the unknown that we sense and the excruciating sense of loss that this foretells.

The talk on depression focuses on the symptoms such as feelings of worthlessness, guilt, lack of pleasure, absence of initiative and of energy, insomnia, and the like less in terms of content than as form or structure. That is, it might be alleged that we all suffer from such symptoms sporadically, but it is their persistence that marks them as indicators of depression. Depression is seen as a problem that causes one to require an expert to determine whether these symptoms "really and truly" add up to what it designates. It is as if depression as a category reflects a kind of tangible thing that we might or might not "have" and that the need to discover this requires consulting someone for verification. That this someone, a medical school graduate, is skilled in such diagnosis, is the comedic upshot of such a vernacular grasp of the category, causing us to imagine lines of subjects waiting to query a facsimile of the Wizard of Oz to ask if the symptoms

Symptoms of depression ***(from Depression Hurts.ca)***

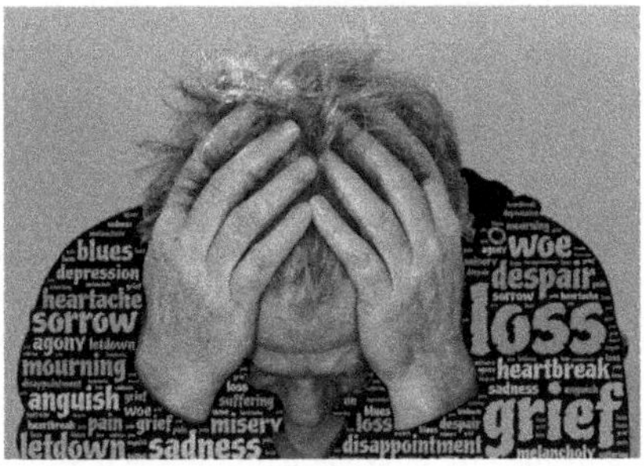

Popular Conceptions

What are the possible symptoms of depression?

Feeling sad, being "depressed," having "dark thoughts" or experiencing difficulty sleeping does not necessarily mean you have depression. For a person to be considered to be suffering from major depressive disorder:

Their symptoms must either be new or must be noticeably worse compared to what they were prior to the episode.

These symptoms also have to persist for most of the day, nearly every day for at least two consecutive weeks.

The episode must also be accompanied by clinically significant distress or impaired functioning.

It is important to discuss all the symptoms you may have with your doctor.

The goal of any treatment is to help you feel more like yourself again so that you are able to enjoy the things you used to. To do so means finding the right treatment to address and alleviate all of your symptoms. Even if you are prescribed medication, this may take some time and may require trying different medications before you find the one that works best. Also, the goal of treatment goes beyond just getting better it is about *staying* better.

Depression is not simply a temporary change in mood or a sign of weakness. It is a real medical condition with many emotional, physical, behavioral, and cognitive symptoms.

Emotional Symptoms

Constant sadness, almost every day

This feeling of sadness can occur for no apparent reason (such as a serious event). It can be intense and feel like there is nothing that will make it go away.

Feeling of worthlessness, of excessive or inappropriate guilt

A depressed person often experiences negative and unrealistic feelings of guilt.

Dark or suicidal thoughts

These ideas can occur frequently during depression. They must be taken very seriously and the person must ask for help right away if they are experiencing such emotions.

Loss of interest or pleasure in favorite activities

This loss of interest may affect all areas of life: from previous hobbies (going to movies, reading, shopping) to everyday activities the person used to enjoy (cooking, doing odd jobs, playing with the children).

Physical Symptoms

Low energy

People with depression often feel low on energy, even when they have not exerted themselves. This depressive fatigue is characterized by the fact that neither rest nor sleep alleviates it.

Psychomotor impairment

Depression may make one feel as if everything is slowed down—slowed speech, thinking, and body movements; increased pauses before answering; speech that is decreased in volume, inflection, amount or variety of content, or muteness may accompany depression.

Aches and pains

Depression can be accompanied by physical pain (headaches, joint pain, stomach pain, and other pains).

Insomnia or its opposite, hypersomnia

Sleep is often broken and unrefreshing. The person often wakes up in the early hours and mental anguish prevents him or her from getting back to sleep. Other cases can include excessive sleep.

Change in weight

Often weight loss or weight gain is a significant sign in diagnosing depression.

Behavioral Symptoms

Change in appetite

Most commonly, appetite is decreased: food seems tasteless and servings too large. Conversely, people sometimes increase their food consumption (especially sweets), which can result in weight gain.

Impression of restlessness

For some people depression makes them feel very agitated and almost jumpy (for example inability to sit still, pacing, hand-wringing, fiddling with clothes or other items, etc.).

Cognitive Symptoms

Difficulty making decisions or focusing

Depression can cause one to experience diminished ability to think or concentrate, or cause one to demonstrate indecisiveness.

If you are experiencing some of the symptoms in the list above and they are affecting your life, do not hesitate to ask for help: you may be suffering from depression.

In this case, seeing a doctor is a crucial step. But, do not overlook the help you can get from those around you—and what you can do to look after yourself.

Only a doctor can diagnose depression

Are you experiencing some of these symptoms?

Are they affecting your life?

Could it be Depression?

Take the test on: http://depressionhurts.ca/en/checklist/

mean that the subject is depressive. All of this speculation depends upon imagining a subject who displays whatever the "disease" is made to require (its symptoms such as self-loathing, inertia, sadness). Yet sadness or immobility is not the reputed issue but their persistence as recurrent matters of orientation for a subject presumed to experience their influence as external constraints upon conduct that seem to cause feelings of self-loathing and indolence. The first step is diagnostic as if deciding whether or not one "has" depression can be determined through expert detection. Yet if depression is a delicately balanced subjective engagement with life and its limits, it seems preposterous to expect a medical school graduate to tune into such a complexity of meaning. This subjective judgment passing itself off as forensic is based upon certain assumptions about the meaning of the category, whether it is transitory or permanent, and what kind of impact it is presumed to have on and for its subject. That the bearer of such a category and its identity sees oneself as determined and as lacking initiative appears to identify the incumbent of the category as experiencing mortification. Regardless of the content, what is required of us is to see in these conditions a particular and singular style of relating to them as a way of being or acting dead. In this sense the subject is seen as performing in life as if a dead person. Depression—even of mortification—then comes alive as a mode of self-affectivity. This reminds us again that any experience, even bodily, is mediated through the signifier as a representation, making depression a signal of anxiety that reflects its ambiguous position in relation to some idea from which it has become separated. Depression is not an affect for which we safely expect medical solutions, even drugs, but the sign of an intricate relationship to life, loss, and the abyssal. Here again we might note Baker's treatment of depression as an attempt to "handle" the problem of perpetual disappointment in life (Baker, 2014) but as an experience that results from overestimating the power of life to deliver what it cannot. It is in this way that what is felt as lost is the innocent expectation of reconciling desire and its destination as final and complete.

In this case the symptoms signal the relation of the one seen as bearing them in the present to some fundamental problem that is covered over through the passage of time by the fabric of the symptom. In other words, what history might such an experience of mortification signal? If such an experience cannot be shared, it might still be imagined by one who bears witness to it through listening to its overtones in words and deeds. What is the expectation that depression offends against and does not name? What is the unspoken interpretive regime that so vividly enters into this representation of oneself? If the depressive appears to orient to the self as mortified in ways that recurrently confirm an experience of feeling dead, this experience might not be accepted at face value as the final word until we explore the possibility that it gives its own kind of pleasure that the jouissance of feeling dead might sustain in certain ways. So if the popular reports enumerate an inventory of self-characterizations, reading through their externality begins to position us in a stronger relation to the underlying discourse towards which they might be trying to find solutions.

Managing the symptoms of sadness or lethargy through drugs is the canonical unreflective relation to conduct that biomedicine also supports and legitimates as the only alternative. Yet we begin to appreciate that a more active plunge into this discourse promises to discover and develop a relationship that can move towards self-knowledge rather than relief of pain. For example, feeling dead could be a way of warding off spirits that arise when the subject takes initiative, and in so doing, risks exposure to evaluation. In such a case feeling dead would be a defense against the anxiety of suffering the ambiguity that always persists in vital action. Being dead might be analogous to a kind of obsessive fear of being seen through, a fear of nakedness often noted in the safe and sound gesture of "playing it close to the vest."

The limited nature of characterizations of depression reveals the conventional wisdom typically used to describe various reputed experiences of sadness, most important, its designation of a medical problem and the practitioner, the doctor, as one who should be consulted. Thus, the paralyzing experience of sadness and the immobility and withdrawal of interest in the world that it seems to show is identified as a terrain for the intervention of medical expertise in addressing one's feelings. If we read this as a common sense version of depression, we can anticipate that in the absence of its theorization, it will be simple to assume its causal history in a neurological or genetic etiology or even some concrete condition such as an external trauma (see Plamper and Lazier 2010 on emotions). Freud ([1917] 1957) upped the stakes in such a desultory conversational history through his contrast of melancholia and mourning by using the "normal prototype" of the death of a loved one as a model that advanced the interpretation of such symptoms as if the funereal sense of loss experienced in being abandoned. Thus, he was able to formulate such symptoms—withdrawal of affect, privatization, anger—as reflections of a response to such abandonment. One question I have been raising throughout this work, and for which there is no final solution, asks: if depression is the name for the experience of being abandoned by meaning, how can we relate to living our life in a meaningful way under such auspices without illusion? How might we engage self and others, and is jouissance possible under such conditions? Is the drive for a meaningful relationship to the abandonment of meaning material for tragedy, comedy, or neither, or then perhaps for another kind of art?

Depression as Abandonment

What the limits of any intended solution to such a question begin to show is that depression mixes anger and sadness, that the sadness in being abandoned is simultaneously converted into anger directed towards the source. But if Freud disclosed this mix so well, I want to reformulate the loss and abandonment not only of a specific other as in grieving but of the belief in life, of meaning, and of the so-called transcendental. What one loses is this belief in the meaning of life, and is abandoned to what Nietzsche called the groundlessness of Being. If it appears that the anger is directed towards life for the betrayal, it could also reveal as its "real" object oneself, because one's basic sense of weakness is perceived as an inability to endure such fundamental ambiguity, seeming to reflect guilt towards one's failure to overcome the experience of lack suggested in such abandonment, the weakness seen as an inability to understand it as a shared relation to fundamental ambiguity rather than as a sign of diminished self-worth and impotence. So the sadness aroused by the loss of meaning and the melancholic relation to one's weakness it elicits could alternatively be treated as a loss to be engaged playfully, not as if one lacks something she could have, but as a condition to be engaged improvisationally as the fundamental ambiguity we all share. In Lacanian, the experience of the lack conveyed metaphorically in the notion of castration needs to be converted into the recognition of the hole in Being.

Taking the caregiver as an example, we note that s/he could react to the dementia as if the loss of a relationship in which s/he is being abandoned by the other, or conversely, the sufferer's reaction to the care could reflect a feeling of being abandoned by the caregiver and/or by life itself, or by the collusion between caregiver and life against the deadening of the sufferer. Such an experience is fundamentally ambiguous even if the loss is treated as unambiguous and factual. Furthermore, whether both caregiver and intimate are angry literally at being abandoned, the caregiver might be angry towards the intimate for deteriorating in a way that "leaves" him or her alone, while the sufferer of dementia can very well be angry at the caregiver for continuing to live and to be engaged.

Beginning from this intuition, I suggest that the cliché of depression used so avidly in everyday life might start from the recognition of such symptoms that in the best (rather than most banal) cases are reconstructions of the complexity of loss assumed to be decisive. For example, if the caregiver's depression is attributed to the experience of losing an intimate and the relationship that such deterioration discloses, then too, this intimate who suffers dementia is not simply feeling the loss of loved ones (that might include the caregiver) but the loss of life and, in its way, of the self. Certainly, this loss of life must include a loss of persons to whom one is attached but we can appreciate its difference from such grieving when we understand its loss as an attachment to life and the commitment and innocence that such belief requires. What might be lost is the passion for life itself, propped up by innocence certainly, and dependent upon the singularity of an archive of sensations and impressions. This enables us to reformulate Freud's experience of abandonment as the underlying force in (so-called) depression in different ways and the dilemma of the caregiver as one of engaging the nuances of such a discourse.

Mourning and Melancholia

In so-called normal speech, the notion of an unconscious makes reference to its motivated, oriented character that can reveal itself in many ways that might be denied or discussed as if irrelevant, for example as in showing disinterest constantly. In such an example, what Lacan calls the "missing encounter" is the opportunity to take up such disinterest as oriented, that is, as the agent's choice rather than an external condition. The intervention can be taken or not, and in its being taken makes transparent the conventionality of the conduct and its oriented character as a matter to engage and track. In terms of an expression, say of fear towards a situation, the conception of the "missed encounter" makes reference to an opening that is not engaged or that is left as a vestige of repetition as if a matter of (what Garfinkel calls) "uninteresting reflexivity" in contrast to seeing it as an opportunity for engaging the representation of fear as matter for discussion, as eventful. To paraphrase Ogden (2012, 24) on the loss of the "object:"

> The melancholic experiences a conflict between, on the one hand, the wish to be alive with the pain of irreversible loss and the reality of death, and on the other hand, the wish to deaden himself to the pain of loss and the knowledge of death. The individual capable of mourning succeeds in freeing himself from the struggle between life and death that freezes the melancholic … the mourner's painful acceptance of the reality of the death of the object is achieved in part because the mourner knows (unconsciously, and, at times, consciously) that his own life, his own capacity for "continuing to live" is at stake.
>
> (Ogden 2012, 29–30)

Here, the caregiver's dilemma is treated as a function of the conflict occasioned by melancholic fixation regarding the prospect of the death of the one cared for in the face of object loss or disappointment, disclosing the melancholic as incapable of mourning, i.e. as unable to face loss and its sense as if deadening oneself to the pain of such loss, and the need to free oneself in order to mourn. This conflict, frequently discussed in the literature (see for example, Abraham and Torok [1987] 1994 and my use of them in Blum 2011a, especially 220–222), pictures mourning as if an advance over melancholia, and so, as a liberation of sorts that promises to counteract depression. Whereas melancholia treats loss as an extinction of the self as a joint death that fixates us on the deprivation in a way that accentuates immobility, in mourning we can imagine living under altered conditions that invite us to honor the significance of the loss in its message to us to incorporate its influence as part of our life and its course. In this sense the lost "object" can remain alive in (our) life, but only if we make a vow to oversee its continued presence as a sign of our indebtedness. This is the problem de Coulanges formulated in our relation to the dead and our ancestors in his classic discussion of Greek religion. This affirms in a different way the relevance of ghosts while confirming that we too will die and will be in no position to guarantee such a legacy. This then reaffirms the relevance of the child as a token of our imaginary sense of a future promise to continue repaying the debt. The jouissance of an investment in life must coexist, as Lacan says, with fantasy insofar as commitment to life depends on the hallucination that we will (can) master time and it is this imaginary conception of a present that requires images of both ghost and the child (Agamben [1978] 1993).

Depression 1: Grief, Paralysis

In the current example of caring for dementia, the conduct of an intimate begins to appear strange as if knowledge has become depersonalized and the figure of one assumed to be known is now rendered unfamiliar. We might say that this is part of the lived experience of the dying intimate, for what had appeared secure in its vitality in life is now alien. It is not just the physical transformation that the dying other seems to be undergoing but the sense of a shared present, of shared togetherness rooted in common interest, that seems to be divisive in ways that separate the sufferer's withdrawal from the caregiver's commitment to the present and future. What is lost is life in the present as a common project.

Assuming the caregiver to be affected by being with someone intimate who is undergoing a radical decline in sentience as reflected in a range of symptoms revealing personal disintegration and a reversal in the capacity for self-composure and self-management that had previously been accepted and secured as stable, we might consider depression in two guises: first, through the experience of the caregiver who is bound to be affected by such a situation, to experience sadness at the other's loss of capacities for independence that had been taken for granted, seeming to grieve the loss of a loved one; second, the loss dovetails with the experience of being overburdened by the absence of reciprocity insofar as the sufferer's responsiveness to the care reflects not the best of the shared history but experiences loss as an absence of recognition by the other that accentuates the lack of mutuality in the strongest sense, as desultory, joyless custodial labor that experiences its own impotence as a force of influence. The sadness of the caregiver is visible on several levels: witness to loss, exposed to a denial of history, taxed by behavior without purpose only to sustain survival and defer an end, tired, possibly abused, invariably disappointed. Here, then, at least for the caregiver, we seem to have all of the ingredients for the symptoms cited of depression in popular culture and diagnostic medicine and therapeutics.

In popular culture and its representations of depression, these symptoms designated are not grounded theoretically, but described from self-reports on feelings and moods that are meant to be self-evident illustrations of depression. In contrast to these surface descriptions, we see that the sense of loss pervading this relationship is an experience of the disappearance of the bond itself and of its substantial function in the life of the caregiver who anticipates remaining with these remains, in this shape as grief.

Depression 2: Reparation

The collective narrative on depression typically posits some movement towards reconciliation as a passage through grief that might overcome paralysis. Though we lack empirical access to the relationship to death as a phenomenon that one can experience as part of the passage of dying, the absence of such "data" still does not mean that the state of mind is unthinkable, for many try to imagine what it is like to experience life as ending. Some of the most vivid illustrations we have come from novelists who create such characters and imagine their relationships in thought and action. Such characterizations of the state of mind of dying as depression always raise the question of the impact of the apparent depression of the dying intimate on the caregiver. What seems to be experienced in caregiving (and possibly reciprocally, in both) is this inability to bridge the experience of dying in a way that can reconcile the relation to loss of each both separately and together.

The problem in trying to reconcile the loss is best represented as the condition of hysteria in that each might say simultaneously and differently, that we are each in our way depressed about dying and yet, you could never know what it is to be me and I could never know what it is to be you. If hysteria begins by aspiring to transgress this border, to say that I am not what you say of me and that I cannot say what I want to say, both the caregiver and the sufferer of dementia are rendered inarticulate by the fact of dying. Here, what is stereotyped as a depressing situation can be seen as an hysterical exchange with each both resisting what is made of them by the other and aspiring to say what cannot be said about this failure. As Lacan suggests of hysteria, each seems blinded by the experience of being objectified by the other, and so, by the inability to say what is essential. Lamentation, not exercised by the grief of loss as reversal of satisfaction and the sadness and fatigue of such behavior, is hysterically attached to loss in ways that begin to make possible poetry and song. If we are truly intimate, I am guilty for continuing to live while you die and you are guilty for leaving me to live and die without you. This can qualify as the saddest song, the mother of all laments.

Here in Hans Keilson's ([1933] 2012, 32–33) novel, the economic distress of a shopkeeper becomes relevant.

> Herr Seldersen sat on the bench for a long time, sunk in thoughts, then he suddenly rouses himself and everything is sharp and clear again the way it was before. He is an old man, life will soon be behind him; he has walked all but the last stretch of the road. But he casts a searching look back over the long path taken so far, and not a single tiny segment escapes his memory. That is my life, he thinks, and all at once the idea comes over him that he will soon have to think about death. But what does death have to do with him? Nothing for the time being, nothing yet… . Who asks after him, who is looking out for him, who? No, no, but now he has to think about it: how to gradually bring his life to a peaceful conclusion. He isn't old yet, he still feels young and vigorous, but the thought comes over him like a soft wind: What if he cannot bring it to a peaceful conclusion?

The recognition of the man that he alone has to work-though and digest death in his own way, without recourse to any other support, produces an intense concentration that seems disturbing to others. Albrecht's death can only preoccupy him in ways that suggest a connection between the conception of mortality and the solitude it imposes as a unique and unshareable experience of the subject. Being alive to death, to risk a pun on this grave matter, imposes the need for concentration that might appear singular and privatized.

In his first novel the Austrian writer Thomas Bernhard ([1963] 2006) created a story in which a medical intern was asked by his supervisor to do him the favor (as part of his training) of visiting and observing the older brother of the supervisor, a decrepit, cantankerous artist living in a remote Austrian village. The resident was instructed to befriend the artist and to observe his behavior in the role of an incognito visitor, eventually reporting back to the supervisor. The narrative of the novel consists of a series of exchanges and reflections in which the relationship between them evolves, centered around the seductive ravings of the artist Strauch. The resident functions much like an observant reflection upon the artist, which is represented in the following selections as if a voice-over running commentary.

> We walk on. He says: "The whole world consists of pointless wastes of strength. I'm waiting for the end now, you know! Just as you're waiting for your end. Just as everyone's waiting for their end … Then: "Vague, always vague! But I don't intend ever to express myself with precision. I can imagine it must be difficult to make anything of these connections, omissions, sins of omission, accumulations, obligations, verdicts … No, I don't demand that! I no longer demand anything. Anything. Nothing from anyone! … A situation like the one in which I find myself is completely unimaginable. Of course, I don't know anything either. That's true. I'm a burden on you … I know your life can't be easy for you either, but it's a good deal easier than mine. "To begin with," he said, "you have all sorts of possibilities. You are able to enthuse about all sorts of things. The most banal things! You develop an array of gifts, of the sort that many people manage to develop, canny people, brutes, and then timid like wallflowers. You can do this and that and the other thing, and your head is stuffed full of all sorts of plans and future directions. All in all, you think you might want to do pretty much anything and have it in your power to do so. You think you're in a circus, and because you're so gifted and so popular, you can do anything in the circus that takes your fancy: any stunts, even the hardest, any tricks, even the meanest. You think you can walk on a tightrope, high over a drop, where the air is already thin … you think you can ride, put your head in the lion's mouth, and take it out when the beast roars … acrobatics … stunts … you think you can do anything, and you also think, and you're completely persuaded of that fact, that you can be the director as well … the circus director: fine, there are no limits, because you see none. It's all unlimited, and that deadly subconscious feeling of being able to turn your hand to absolutely anything … till one day your first idea comes to you, and then a second, a third, and a fourth … one after another … finally hundreds and thousands, thousands of ideas: those are the painters, the newspapermen, the prison wardens and the prisoners, the policemen, the philosophers … heir, cow, tail, minister, director, you understand … till you end up not being convinced by anything … that's what it is … Because you have your moments of this and that, and no character … how soon everything turns into nothing, unemployed, unskilled, mad, unemployable, manifesting the signs of idiocy … But all that's just a point of view," he said, "no deeper and no less deep than the crassest error."
>
> (212–213, Bernhard's ellipses)

To concede that what he says is just a "point of view" is an important concession after his rant, for he acknowledges that even his nihilism must suffer the chronic and apparently irreparable contradiction that haunts life in the prosaic shape of relativism, but more deeply as the two-sided relationship to the unknown that is our fate, acting as if we know that about which we inevitably remain ignorant.

> One day you get home, and you know that from now on you have to pay for everything, and from that moment on you're old and dead. One day, everything is finished, though life itself might go on for a while. You're dead, and beauty and whatever happiness is and wealth, everything has withdrawn from you forever.
>
> (336–338)

This might be the moment that recognizes life as betrayal and that inspires both indifference and impatience, and yet that reveals waiting as necessary in two senses, almost as a corporeal drive, and as something to be seen through as the "pointless wastes of strength" it seems to be. Here, what the artist recognizes is that any antidote to boredom is a lure and nothing more, a further extension of the waiting that occurs as inevitable. As such, life as a continuous project can only appear as doing time, as waiting. Thus, if solitude could be the common fate suffered at end-of-life, as a glimpse of nihilism that aging can bring to life for its wide-awake subject, one way to understand age-related dementia is to explore what the singularity of persons might contribute to such an adjustment (see Blum 2011a; 2013).

This aporia comes alive in Anita Brookner's (2009) novel when a lonely aged person, on the occasion of his relative's death and her bequest of property to him, recognizes that it still makes no difference.

> He would no more sentimentalize past attachments, no longer trace the memory of the old house, a line had come to be drawn between past and present, or rather between past and whatever time remained to him. That that time would be grave he had no doubt: without attachments he would have to face it alone. Those strangers in whom he had put his trust might turn away, indifferent to his plight, and he would have only his own thoughts for company.
>
> (96)

> The image came to him again, as did the conviction that he must change, if he was to make his remaining time tolerable.
>
> (121–122)

> He was not sorry to see his past for what it was but it had one morbid and disturbing effect: he no longer slept well. Without the comforting illusion of a context he could not ignore the fact that he was on his own and had always been so, and that sleep was no longer his refuge. He would wake suddenly, not knowing where he was, knowing only that he was adrift. In the hours of

> daylight he could dismiss his night fears, knowing that they were the baleful signs of old age, that they foreshadowed a death, which, though not immanent, was inevitable. For that reason he made strenuous efforts to live in the present, and sometimes almost succeeded. But the present was a poor thing without company. Which brought him back to his resolution to make things new while he still had a chance to do so.
>
> (140)

> These memories of the past … did little to assuage his habitual melancholy. Nor did the realization that with the disappearance of this connection he was now truly free of the past. He would not regret this. In attempting to see himself as others saw him he also saw that he had become the character he thought suitable: appearance had become reality. He was respectable; he had nothing to hide. But having nothing to hide also meant an inner emptiness, and a predisposition to any fantasy that might fill that onerous gap.
>
> (188)

The necessity for productive life to be blocked and repressed, thoroughly immersed in its projects that fortify it in any present, means that the experience of loss that might emerge is the loss of one's life in ways different than what is reputed as the depression of the caregiver.

The overburdened caregiver then has to imagine the experience of loss suffered in the refrain of one who experiences the end-of-life as if a lament on ending. The poetic refrains of each character in these novels seems to function as ways of making the strangeness of death (the relation to the unknown that it manifests) somewhat transparent in these renditions of familiar experiences, and so, of making anonymity intimate by virtue of representing the whole prosaically. This is done by taking up the cliché of dying and its assortment of significations and depersonalizing them in situations as reflective engagements of characters condemned to ruminate on such conventions. Thus, the novel twists and reconfigures these relationships in ways that aspire to make the strange (death and its terror) intimate (palpable, familiar) through a method of making what is familiar (and intimate), such as the cliché of death and depression, strange and uncanny in stories.

Depression 3: Bearing Witness

The dilemma of anyone exposed to the impending death of an intimate, the problem of how to comport oneself in ways that are true to the experience and not simply formulaic, means that the temptation to depersonalize the relationship as if a professional transaction guided by asymmetrical structures and expectations needs to be overcome. The difference between the living and the dying must not be made essential just as the closeness between the living and dying needs to be moderated: neither/nor guides the relationship between intimacy (of caregiver and other) and anonymity (of the different experience of each). Though we are different (I live while you die), we are still connected as intimates: though similar (as such connected beings), your dying differentiates you from my living in ways that make our situation enigmatic. Aside from the possible experience of pain, what can the subject of dementia be thinking, and how do the scrambled words bear upon such thoughts? Here, we are invited to imagine the relationship to death as a course of action being articulated by one undergoing it. That sense of death must include not only a glimpse of its apparent irrationality and absurdity (even as a "rational" physical event) but also its ludicrous character as a state of awareness that information cannot relieve. Thus, the paralyzing ambiguity of the relation of biology to life is glimpsed without satisfaction. Certainly science and social work can give no assistance here: at best they can point to experiences such as pain, incoherence, or distress but not to the representation of such experiences in the thinking that dwells upon its encounter. Here again we confront the uncanny aura of the expiry date as a label pinned to the human forehead.

Further, this conundrum is not due simply to uncertainty stimulated by diagnostic mysteries but to the experience of having to share the "burden" of imagining the end-of-life. This suggests that the very enigma of care tends to be disregarded as anything but a technical problem of service delivery or provisioning when the sufferer of dementia is treated as neurologically incapacitated because this leaves the caregiver with little opportunity for intervention in a creative way, forcing such a subject to resign to custodial care in order to survive the situation. It is not simply the case that the biomedical model is reductive in diagnosing and treating age-related dementia, but by inflating hyperbolically this view of the subject, it tends to reduce the caregiver to a passivity insofar as the view of the other as condemned to somatic incapacities is a fundamental constraint upon action. Care is trapped between the twin temptations of resignation and the tendency to act out that simply recoils against bureaucratic treatment, responses that result from an inability to conceive of an impersonal relationship to suffering that is not depersonalized. But more fundamentally care is positioned between the desire to speak the truth about impending death and the fear it plainly arouses, and the need to be supportive towards the intimate who is experiencing this futureless future.

The reflective ruminations of the characters in these novels as situated by the writer is dramatized when we compare them with the denial of death expressed in many other characters such as the anxiety disclosed in the picture of his mother developed by David Rieff, the son of Susan Sontag. The depression of the caregiver comes alive in his story of the support he gave her during the last period of her struggle with cancer and what he and others sensed as her inevitable movement towards death: "In retrospect … I realize that, obsessed with death as she was, this positive denial was at a deep level the denial of death itself" (2008, 92). The son's quandary occurs as a result of his sensitivity to Sontag's attempt to deny death because of her hold on life and her aspiration, of course, to stay vital and maintain her productivity.

> So, again and again, I look at her life's trajectory and see the future tense elbowing out the present. And yet surely the only way to even remotely come

> to terms with death is to live in the present… . Anyway that is the way it was for my mother. She would not contemplate extinction until the last month of her life… . Which was her right. I'm sure of that. What I'm far less sure of is whether I did the right thing in going along with and in fact doing what I could to abet her in her refusal to contemplate the prospect that … she would die of cancer… . This is probably one variant of … "the loved one's dilemma" … Did I do the right thing? Could I have done more? Or proposed an alternative? Or been more supportive? Or forced the issue of death to the fore? Or concealed it better?
>
> (202–221)

Rieff's concern follows from his desire to support his mother's conception of her future even as he recognizes its denial of the truth, positioning him in this space of contradiction, wanting to do the best by and for her in a way that honors the inevitability of the situation: "My mother had always thought of herself as one whose hunger for truth was absolute. After her diagnosis, the hunger remained, but it was life and not truth that she was desperate for. I hope I did the right thing in trying to give it to her, but I will never be sure" (102).

Rieff's dilemma is characteristic of any caregiver, but in this situation his parent's aspiration to immortality was a function of her embrace of an Enlightenment imaginary of productivity and mastery that envisioned her perpetuity, resting on her belief in being special in such a way, which made fearing a loss in death of all she thought herself to be an unbearable experience. Indeed, Sontag's idealization of science and rationality and her mechanical addiction to herself without irony both repels him and reconfigures his loyalty and love:

> I knew that for her the physical agony she was undergoing … was only bearable because of this hope and that therefore my task had to be to help her as best I could to go on believing that she would survive… . Never for a moment, during the course of my mother's illness, did I think that she could have "heard" that she was dying.
>
> (104)

> When my mother was at her most disconsolate, she would often say, "This time for the first time in my life, I don't feel special."
>
> (85)

The equality and homogeneity inflicted on us by the inevitability of death always threatens to erase our sense of being special, of being and/or having a self. This fear reaffirms the tension we noted in Lacan's conception of the division between the experience of death as absolute (singular, for me in particular) and as relative (universal and inevitable) for Other. Certainly Sontag's fanatic self-absorption and displaced commitment to reason as science could only heighten this anxiety.

Note again that while the dementia sufferer might be lost to the caregiver, the loss of an intimate, the lost object for this sufferer is possibly imaginable as life, or more prosaically, as the self itself. The dementia sufferer does not just lose the caregiver but loses life and the self and the sense of singularity inescapably bound to it. This is what the Lear effect could suggest. In other words, the sufferer of dementia is engaged by the loss of the self and the melancholic fixation this evokes. If dementia sufferer and caregiver disclose two different voices in this discourse, two different approaches to the "object" of death and its imaginative structure, or two different senses of the lost object, then what notion of loss binds these differences or holds them together? Such a question comes to view for theorizing and for the voice of an art that can recognize both its distance from this interaction at present and the togetherness disclosed in how everyone is bound by the common problem of loss and the need to develop a healing relation to its inevitability.

The literature on mourning and melancholia reveals that the capacity to continue to live is at stake and the caregiver must be taught to recognize that this very well might be the problem that lies behind the scrambled hallucinatory text of the dementia sufferer. Thus, a novelist, for example, stands to model the practice of mourning as a reflective engagement with the sense of loss of self in the contemplation of death. Unlike biomedical intended solutions that treat the very notion of a self as a case of bewitchment, ignorance, succumbing to the illusion of "ghost in the machine" and the like, views of mourning do not accuse false consciousness or counsel renunciation of the self but instead accept as Real the struggle of life and death of the self as the drive to overcome one's deadening, knowing full well that death is forthcoming. Could we venture that the need and desire to overcome deadening is the primordial problem (and priority) of the human subject?

The self is then divided by the tension between knowledge of death and the need to overcome its tendency to produce deadening in order to live. That the knowledge of death always promises to deaden us reiterates the force of the nihilist voice throughout life, and makes any resistance to it appear illogical, soft-hearted, cowardly, subjective, and targets for the various taunts that nihilism directs at the faint-hearted in order to energize its own testosterone level under trying circumstances. Thus, transforming the division in death itself between its character as mortal extinction and end of biological life, and this sense of deadening in life as a second death, is practiced in the mournful and comic action that takes upon itself the drive to resist the demand to deaden one's own life while knowing full well that life is bound to die.

In this respect, I can imagine the use of different and varied materials from sources other than medical science as ingredients for a curriculum designed not simply to have anthropological value for expanding horizons, but as a method for intervening in our silent and obscene collective monologue regarding death and for handling the anxieties of anticipating its unknown ramifications (on this discourse see Blum 2011a, especially 183–234; 2011b; Chapter 7 of this volume; Blum 2014; see also Chapter 5 in this volume). I suggest that we begin thinking of the ravings of the dementia text as such a script and of the sense of helplessness in relation to such a speech as part of the force and inscrutability of the discourse. In this way, I can contemplate such a program as a first step for creating a sense of the conversion of melancholic paralysis into a stronger and mournful relationship to loss and lack that the reflective anticipation of death brings to mind. Here, Lacan's comment on bearing witness displayed earlier seems pertinent.

Yet we see how Bataille's position speaks as if one suddenly confronts life as a betrayal when what he calls the intimate connection to oneself is made dramatic and transparent, as if, freed suddenly from the preoccupation of work, activity, and what he calls the project, from being occupied by seeing oneself as what he calls a thing, and suddenly coming face-to-face with the Real, face-to-face with the There-is, and its character as Nothing: "No one knew it was there when it was; it was overlooked in favor of real things: death was one real thing among others. But death suddenly shows that the real society was lying" (Bataille [1973] 1989, 47). Note again how unlike Bataille, Lacan treats this not as betrayal at all, because life has made clear as its ever-present connotation the inevitability of death, meaning that all life, in his words, is a detour from this intuition and not a betrayal at all but a defense against its recognition. Nevertheless the anger in expressions attributed to dementia sufferers can be understood as reactions to their discovery of the truth of death and the recognition of their difference from those still "taken in" by life and its lie. Both Bataille and Lacan can recognize the anger in mortal responses to the experience of life as betrayal. This remains a test for the reflective one, to overcome this anger.

Addiction to Life

The denial of death is needed to enhance the capacity to live life in any present just as the desire to live needs to be cultivated in ways that can help repress the thought of death. This suggests that the repression of death is sustained by the desire to discover and attach oneself to some worldly preoccupation in a way that requires life to need and value what Kenneth Burke (1957) calls "equipment for living" by virtue of its being a method for putting aside the thought of death. This makes the repression of death equivalent to what is called in competitive sports a "performance enhancing" drug, akin to an addiction. Investment in the relevance of the worldly preoccupation that depends upon repressing the thought of death and our primordial solitude is analogous to the way in which a drug enhances our capacity to perform at life. In this way solitude can identify an orientation to the evanescence of worldly attachments that is in between the affective investment in the attachment as if conclusive and definitive and an awareness of the limits of this gesture. What Gadamer ([1993] 1996) glosses, and only comes to view in the contribution of Lacan, is how the inversion of the repression of death as the motivated attachment to some preoccupation has to be invested with jouissance or a degree of affect that can sustain it.

Therefore we might suggest that the in-between status of dementia, deriving from the subject's necessary intermediacy between the commitment to life and the intuition of mortality (between the absorption of the finite and the specter of infinite perplexity that haunts the finite), is exactly what loosens the hold of life upon subject and simultaneously opens the subject to the solitude of mortality.

Jouissance tells us that we not only can enjoy the worldly preoccupation by repressing the thought of death but that we can enhance the performance of its life by endowing it with the eroticism accompanying a playful engagement with its contingency. The caregiver needs to understand the connection between the conduct of the intimate who suffers dementia and the loosening of the hold of life that produces at this time the awareness of the limits of mortality as registered in the speech that appears crazed and hallucinatory. This begins to develop the relationship of mourning and allows us to deepen our inquiry into care.

Passing Time

I suggest in this situation a conception of the dementia sufferer as a social actor challenged by the need to work out in specific ways a struggle with the nihilist and the return of the repressed as part of the reflective "doubling" of an internal conversation. Thus, the caregiver could be educated to deal with this as a witness rather than exclusively as a provider or custodian. Fixation upon the brain and its degeneration risks distracting the caregiver from such a position or role. One problem is that the caregiver is also subject to such tension—the inability to imagine death—and must share the suffering of this "problem" as part of shared being. The deficit in imagination that both caregiver and sufferer disclose is not a loss but a lack that can be reshaped from available resources. The caregiver needs to change in this direction as a way of working-through this struggle on his/her own as well as listening to the dementia sufferer. What *is* worked out is a problem that is common and the need for shared witnessing. The problem is nothing other than the desire to imagine the unimaginable and to put it into words.

If the idea of the "end-of-life" has weight as a phenomenological experience to which we orient, rather than as an indifferent mark, then the experience of impending death and its inevitability should be part of the speech and conduct of such a subject, even indirectly as part of the "text" of the subject, even in ways of which one might be unaware. In this respect, caregivers would need to track such implications by learning to read and hear the talk for such overtones.

I have suggested that if the hallucinatory talk of dementia seems like word salad, there remains an intelligibility in the speech, but an intelligibility in its problem-solving and not simply in the way it conforms to causal description (to descriptions of its material or efficient causes). Yet I have also suggested that neurology, as rational as it might appear, is guided by its own exclusions, dreams, and delusions, by the very kind of unconscious dynamic that it denies or forecloses in the diagnosis of dementia and of the caregiver.

In the clearer idiom of Wittgenstein, depression is part of a language game that does a variety of exclusions and holds such gestures in abeyance as if extraneous and unspoken. The game is based upon a certain picture of the relation of language to the world.

In this chapter I have tried to disclose, after Freud, the unspoken problem of this game and its players who I formulated as trying to produce solutions to the experience of loss and, as suggested, to the abandonment of meaning, as an experience that creates the possibility of a collection of diverse adjustments and its mix of sadness and anger. This is the Real that posits the notion of an excess or surplus of connotations beyond the word depression, pointing to the subject's engagement by such ambiguity and the need to act under the condition of its limitation, or under the auspices of what Plato called the final cause. This leads me to ask: how can we begin to overcome the temptation to act out and devalue life that this hysterical exchange might influence? How might we begin to find our bearings in a world where, to paraphrase Deleuze ([1995] 2005), influence is a remote possibility? This is an open question and our opener for conversation and research.

Conclusion

In this sense I approach death as a conundrum, always present and held in abeyance as an uncanny register occasionally glimpsed, in ways unsettling and needing to be put to rest. The repression of death is a thought that must be quieted if we are to be engaged in our lives. I conceive of life as a problem-solving situation and the "problem" as the need to expel, while yet honoring, the temptation to be exercised by the enigmatic question of our mortal limits. In this work I keep asking how, given death, we could live and act, as if this is a perennial though "sub-textual" problem not only for dementia and its caregivers but for many others than the aged, lonely, and forlorn. I have sought to track the discourses, instabilities, limits, and problem-solving that our relation(s) to mortality raises to an imaginative eye and to develop ways and means of healing indecision, resignation, sadness and anger, fear and trembling in the face of such fundamental ambiguity. To this end I have plunged into a discourse that we are part of and inherit, such as the commonplace doxa on depression and the various opinions expressed about its characteristics.

References

Abraham, Nicolas and Maria Torok. (1987) 1994. *The Shell and the Kernel: Renewals of Psychoanalysis, Volume I.* Edited and translated by Nicolas T. Rand. Chicago: University of Chicago Press.

Agamben, Giorgio. (1978) 1993. *Infancy and History: The Destruction of Experience.* Translated by Liz Heron. London: Verso.

Baker, Annie. 2014. *The Flick.* New York: Theatre Communication Group.

Bataille, Georges. (1973) 1989. *Theory of Religion.* Translated by Robert Hurley. New York: Zone Books.

Bernhard, Thomas. (1963) 2006. *Frost: A Novel.* Translated by Michael Hoffman. New York: Vintage.

Blum, Alan. 2011a. *The Grey Zone of Health and Illness.* Bristol, UK: Intellect Press.

——. 2011b. "Life, Death and the In-Between: The Duck/Rabbit and the Face of the Clown." In *Spectacular Death: Interdisciplinary Perspectives on Mortality and (Un) representability*, edited by Tristanne Connolly, 21–41. Bristol: Intellect Press.

——. 2013 "Aging as a Social Form: The Phenomenology of the Passage." *Journal of Medical Humanities* 35: 19–36.

——. 2014. "Guide(s) for the Perplexed: Science and Literature as Equipment for Living." *Philosophy and Rhetoric* 48 (1): 54–72.

——. 2016. *The Lived Experience of the Dying Body*. London: Routledge.

Brookner, Anita. 2009. *Strangers*. New York: Random House.

Burke, Kenneth. 1957. *The Philosophy of Literary Form: Studies in Symbolic Action.* Berkeley, CA: University of California Press.

Chandler, James. 2007, "On the Face of the Case: Lord Jim and the Sentimental Novel." In *On the Case: Critical Inquiry* 33 (4): 837–864.

Deleuze, Gilles. (1995) 2005. *Pure Immanence: Essays of a Life, Second Edition.* Translated by Anne Boyman. New York: Zone Books.

Freud, Sigmund. (1917) 1957. "Mourning and Melancholia." In *Volume 11, On Metapsychology: The Theory of Psychoanalysis*, translated by James Strachey, 245–268. London: Penguin.

Gadamer, Hans-Georg. (1993) 1996. *The Enigma of Health: The Art of Healing in a Scientific Age*. Translated by John Gaiger and Nicholas Walker. Stanford: Stanford University Press.

Garfinkel, Harold. 1967. *Studies in Ethnomethodology.* Englewood Cliffs, NJ: Prentice Hall.

Keilson, Hans. (1933) 2012. *Life Goes On.* New York: Farrar, Strauss and Giroux.

Lingis, Alphonso. 2000. "To Die With Others." *Diacritics* 30 (3): 106–113.

Nancy, Jean-Luc. 2000. *Being Singular-Plural.* Stanford: Stanford University Press.

McHugh, Peter. 2005. "Shared Being, Old Promises, and the Joint Necessity of Affirmative Action." *Human Studies* 28: 129–156.

Ogden, Thomas H. 2012. "Freud's 'Mourning and Melancholia' and the Origins of Object Relations Theory." In *Creative Readings: Essays on Seminal Analytic Works*, 14–33. London: Routledge.

Plamper, Jan, and Benjamin Lazier. 2010. "Introduction: The Phobic Regimes of Modernity." *Representations* 110 (1): 58–65.

Rieff, David. 2008. *Swimming in a Sea of Death: A Son's Memoir.* New York: Simon and Schuster.

11 Tragedy and Comedy

Introduction

This chapter tries to bring together the notions of fate and destiny by treating fate as the need to invest meaning in oneself as this takes shape as a symptom that is both inescapable as a particular style of existence that operates like a signature and as an incentive for more, for the desire to rise above such a trademark and be innovative in relation to this inheritance. I use T.J. Clark's analyses of the paintings of Pouisson to see his art as an intended solution to this division between life and death that he advances through the idea of an "awakening." I treat fate as the way the contingencies of a life become legible as the façade of a history and life and destiny as the inescapable narrative that any such conclusion can fertilize (Clark 2006). This opens the door to a speculation on how a comedic relationship to mortality and its dependency on an unknown future, and the uses made of us in the hands of others can serve as a contrast to the pathos of tragedy and its foretelling of a nomadic passage through the corridors of eternity.

The Gift

As I mentioned earlier, Gadamer ([1993] 1996, 156) tells us that the gift of Prometheus to humankind for which Zeus punished him was not fire, as typically thought, but the capacity to forget death. This gift was developed by Aeschylus' reading of the myth:

> The myth relates how Prometheus stole fire from heaven and taught mankind to work with it. But Aeschylus presents the story in a way which makes the theft of fire almost incidental. Prometheus glories in having performed the greatest possible service to man—who had been left so poor and defenseless by Zeus—by depriving him of the knowledge of his own death.

Amnesia is a peculiar gift: The truth is sacrificed and humans need to live with false beliefs in order to survive. The truth would kill them, annihilate their spirit. But then the moral seems: repress the truth for a better life. I suggest that the world of tragedy is the world of this "better life" as a world without the truth that the repression tries to banish, and that comedy lives not outside this world but within it as one kind of therapy or antidote to its limits as part of its effort to develop a surrogate art that can replace this lost "truth." Then if the truth evokes a sense of totality and its necessity *and* ambiguity, this two-sided Grey Zone might both require and repel knowledge of death because the thought of our mortality, even if vexatious, must be factored into our relationship to the world. So if we never really possessed this truth but only had it in an external way, what Prometheus represses is the opportunity to learn about this truth in a strong way, of learning about it and how to engage it. What we can learn about this engagement with the presence of death is how we need to discriminate between the fatalistic and inspirational dimensions of our inevitable destination. We see that as any repression this one is not a total erasure because it leaves this truth both present and absent or makes it into what we can call an absent presence or a present absence.

For many, the truth that is sacrificed is somewhat like a poetic conception of the world that is capable of bearing the ambiguity of indeterminate or opaque events and notions, resembling what is often seen as an elaboration of the sacred. So it appears as if Prometheus says to humans that he will dispense some medication to them that will allow them not to worry about that which they cannot take the measure of and that will only disperse and distract them. It is as if Prometheus says: look chums, just forget poetry, meaning, and all of that stuff that will drive you crazy because it will open up a quagmire or swamp that you will hallucinate as a Grey Zone; here, I'll give you some medicine called the antidote of repression. It's a gift and forget about repaying me!

In previous work (Blum 2011) I used the anthropologist Malinowski to illustrate how the sacred could serve as the intimation of a problem-solving situation, implicitly identifying death and illness as indicators of the fundamental ambiguity of meaning for anyone and everyone, making the problem a situation of action that requires (Kenneth Burke would say) sizing this up and coming to terms with it. That is, given fundamental ambiguity how do we handle its problem in a wholesome way? In the book I said:

> The enigma of both disease and death, according to Malinowski, is connected to their appearing as conditions that are ambiguous, both natural and inexplicably related to forces not necessarily of the same order, apprehended in a "hazy emotional mist" as if both natural and supernatural forces that are related to conditions assumed linked to the singularity of a person and his/her destiny. At the most elemental level, the Grey Zone of health and illness appears as the conundrum of such mysterious causality, how its impersonality as both natural and Other can only be remedied by technique supplemented by prayer.
>
> (Blum 2011, 49)

In line with a notable but often disregarded convention of inquiry this suggests that the sacred has to be seen as more than aesthetic and ethical but as functional in Simmel's sense, designed to solve the problem of connecting us to the world in the face of its fundamental ambiguity. Thus, we can begin to see the need for the sacred, its character as equipment for living in Kenneth Burke's sense, and to appreciate the sacred as a method or means rather than as simply content or doctrine in Marshall McLuhan's sense, the sacred being a medium that massages us in this situation of perplexity. If we require the sacred or its analogue to handle problems that are intractable, when the sacred is withdrawn we still must handle fear and trembling, that is, anxiety and its affects.

I suggest that what Malinowski means is implied in a tradition of inquiry that pictures the human subject befuddled and bewildered by the ineffable and complex world and at a loss to explain natural forces that seem inscrutable. In this situation the subject views a condition such as death as akin to the natural cycle of birth and rebirth undergone by what is regarded as nature and its processes, or by seeing disease as analogous to the inevitable cycle of growth and deterioration of natural things. Such a subject, to paraphrase Vico, might be driven to poetry in order to analogically represent such unknown forces and processes. Here poetry is not meant as the genre in contrast to prose, but as a figure for the spark that ignites a spirited engagement with meaning and its resonances, somewhat like the notion of desire. I am using poetry to stand in for the desire to engage the figurativeness of language without guilt. This kind of engagement with the world could be resigned and fatalistic as is often reputed and if a compensation for ignorance, will also be seen as destined for extinction with the advance of knowledge. Yet, we want to consider whether such a disposition towards the world might still be necessary and desirable in the society ruled by so-called knowledge, the society we conceive as the world of tragedy. Thus, my simple thesis is that tragedy both expels such narrative desire and surreptitiously registers anxiety over its absence regularly and recurrently in the affective structure of modern life, and that this absence is often experienced in part as the incentive that drives us towards comedy. Further, as a program for theory and research we propose strategies for analyzing the repression of such desire in everyday life and to develop avenues for improvising with experimental strategies for recovering its weight as part of a strategy for enhancing the value of life for many.

In this chapter I begin by using the cliché of the repression of death and of the sacred as a condition for the advance of knowledge as a way into the discourse that distinguishes, opposes, or aligns tragedy and comedy. Thus, in repressing death, Prometheus might be said to repress jouissance as a way of inhabiting the abyss and of converting it into a scene of seductiveness: by inflicting this upon us he forces us to live life under the rule of our symptoms as if the best we might do is symptom management.

The Extinction and Revival of Poetry in Tragedy

If the world of tragedy risks expelling the desire to theorize while yet maintaining a vestige of it in the genre of tragedy, this makes tragedy an important opportunity to see the tension in theorizing that is played out in the contrast of tragedy and comedy, since both tragedy and comedy are parts of a discourse on subjectivity. By withdrawing the desire to theorize and the link that mediates the relation of subject to natural forces, we abandon the subject to a kind of passivity where to paraphrase Socrates, one can only weep and wail and hold their wounded parts in grief. Following Seth Benardete's version of tragedy as a picture of the world in which the sacred has been withdrawn, the world that Prometheus thought he saved with the gift of repressing death, we can identify the wasteland (so to speak) because the world of tragedy seems a world where people are connected by a language with bare bones, devoid of any sense of resonance, vagueness, and open texture, an environment pictured as organized by a model of contractual relations between monads, mutually oriented but rule governed and lacking resources for more, the world where everyone seems compelled in the face of ambiguity to participate in rancorous exchanges. So the withdrawal of the sacred glosses the real matter which is the withdrawal of the desire for the elemental nature of representation as disclosed in the art of theorizing. We might suggest that the withdrawal of the sacred amounts to withdrawing the capacity for dialogue over the question of what dream might best satisfy our need for such as equipment for living?

David Foster Wallace implies in his afterword to the novel by David Markson (*Wittgenstein's Mistress*, 1988), that we might imagine a subject inhabiting the world of the *Tractatus* as a normal and taken-for-granted environment. The novel, he says, is "an imaginative portrait of what it would be like *actually to live* in the sort of world the logic and metaphysics of Wittgenstein's *Tractatus* posits. The sort of world started out for Wittgenstein to be logical heaven. It ends up being… a metaphysical hell" (Wallace 1988, 252). In this case, think of the world of tragedy as somewhat like living out the *Tractatus*. What is withdrawn with the sacred is then the capacity for theorizing, reflected here as the desire for the elemental.

I have called by the name of travesty this type of methodological intervention that Peter McHugh and I used over time and this kind of thought experiment has been a feature of our work over the years as a means of interrupting the usage and discourses and forcing their instabilities to become observable and accessible to analysis. If travesty reiterates Wittgenstein's reminder that we do not ask for what belongs with a phraseology but for the wish it expresses that I amended as the hope and the fear, we can ask for the hope and fear expressed by the world of tragedy (but only) by virtue of our desire to theorize. We are interested in how the phraseology shows what must exceed it in the unstated hopes and fears it expresses (the relation Georg Simmel depicts between life (which is akin to phraseology), and more than life (as the wish any phraseology can be seen on inspection to express). In looking at and past the phraseology we seem perverted since we alter the natural uses of the phrase to see through it. It is not that we take what someone says and use it against them but in perverting it we read it by inverting its surface to see its concealed purposes in relation to its desire to realize some ideal, we sexualize the phraseology of the text by seeing the jouissance it expresses, its hopes and fears. Travesty imagines the type of actor that must be assumed by a theory and its parameters for inhabiting its world as if the subject hypothesized is ruled by the categories, conditions, and courses of action implied that are specified by the theory as its requirements. This is the gesture of exaggeration in travesty.

This subject is akin to what Schutz called the puppet that is assumed to embody the theory in practice and to live according to its background as if an environment of conditions for action. This view allowed Garfinkel (1967) to read every theory not simply as an abstract text but as a set of instructions for bringing an action to fruition in ways that invariably expose its limits and remainder.

In the world of tragedy, Oedipus as the personification of the public man and his immersion in externals can only be disrupted by the intimation that the unknown exceeds what he can make of it, that his "who" exceeds his "what." Oedipus is furious at Tiresias for reminding him that there is more there than meets the eye. Again David Foster Wallace on Markson's novel: "One of the things that so putatively tortured Wittgenstein in the 20 years between the *Tractatus* and the *Investigations* was that a logically atomistic metaphysics admits exactly of nothing of ethics or moral value or questions of what it is to be human. It's history that Wittgenstein the person cared about what made things good or right or worthwhile" (259). That is, the actor implicitly projected by such a framework when it is conceived as an environment of action, must behave without conceptions that seem necessary and desirable for living a life in the context that the theory stipulates as its conditions. It is such a view of travesty that enables us to appreciate how the gift of Prometheus created a world with very important elements excluded and so *made* the actor into one vulnerable to the lack of such resources. Travesty exacerbates the course of action of the subject in order to expose the Grey Zone between the symbolic order (the theory) and the Real that always must materialize as the spectacle of the actor's need to dispose of ambiguity. We use the figure of the algorithm as an irony designed to bring to view the inescapable remainder that haunts any action as its surplus, implicitly mocking the single-minded faith in the stepwise description of an action as ideal. In this way travesty recovers the praxiological element of action.

Here now I repeat the exchange between Prometheus and the chorus from Aeschylus:

> P: I stopped mortals from seeing death in front of them
> C: What remedy did you find for this disease?
> P: I settled blind hope in them
> C: You gifted mortals with a great benefaction.
> P: Besides this I gave them fire
> C: And now mortals who live for a day have flame-faced fire?
> P: Yes, and from it they will learn many arts
>
> (Aeschylus 1956, 148–150)

Benardete says:

> "Mortals once saw death as their lot in front of them; they could not have simply foreseen the day of their death … for then Prometheus would not have been compelled to give them blind hopes; he would have only had to take this faculty away. Prometheus made death invisible (Hades). The pre-Promethean

> situation of men was the constant awareness of death, and as this made any activity based on future expectations impossible, which is the presumption of any productive art, Prometheus had to remove men's oppressive sense of their own mortality before the arts could become useful. Mortals are ephemeral, according to the Chorus; they live in the light of day in which they once saw themselves as only mortal. But Prometheus' gift of fire, coupled with blind hopes, means the replacement of this natural light by artificial light, whose purpose is precisely to conceal the original horizon within which men live. The price paid for the arts is blindness.…The Chorus believe that to see death before one's eyes is a disease, and that Prometheus benefited men in setting blind hopes in them.
>
> (Benardete 2000, 115)

Before tragedy in the pre-Promethean world we have a situation in which we are attuned to mortality and its frightening resonance and at the same time, can engage this premonition with the support of the sacred. Yet the chorus treats this as a diseased situation and the sacred as medicine, making Prometheus' gift seem the best antidote for this disease by helping humans cure themselves. In other words, repression is better medicine than the sacred, or repressing meaning is better medicine in our kind of world than focusing upon meaning! However, if we make a deal to eliminate death from our horizon, and we pay this debt by giving up on the sacred, we still need some armor to engage life with all of its turbulence. Here we have to understand the Grey Zone as originating in Prometheus' gift: on the one hand, its offer of relief of death, and on the other hand, its infliction of blindness. We might push this further for it is much like medicine: the symptom is managed but the underlying condition remains. So fear of death could be a symptom of an underlying and intractable anxiety that is ineradicable, i.e. inevitable. This is the relationship to the unknown. We could say that Prometheus allows humans to lay this anxiety aside by making death invisible; but it is bound to reappear in the return of the repressed. Could we say that the fear of death is like a phobic reaction to the enigma of the meaning of life?

Social life and its symbols and requirements including the superego, norms, and whatnot, not only mark the point where loss, expectation, deprivation, dispossession, ambition, and all of the mundane affects and the anxieties they cover over begin to percolate, but by virtue of this moment, identifies a space where defenses and resistances needed for fortification must emerge. It is necessary to keep the thought of death in the background and this is done by converting our sense of failure and limit into virtues: to compensate through worldly preoccupations and to carry on. What we feel as lost is actually the sense of innocence that fortified us against an obsession about death and so the capacity to rekindle such innocence in our present and its preoccupations. Such innocence is practiced in language in part, as the disciplined poetry intrinsic to the practice of theorizing. We want to regain the innocence that marked our participation in the sacred.

The gift is curious for it is also a kind of punishment. Humans acquire the productive arts, hopes and aspirations, a sense of the future and the significance of their present in time, and correlative with this gift, a blindness towards their situation and its mortal limits. So in a strange way humans get knowledge, which is what the productive arts amount to, a capacity to symbolize, calculate, appraise, represent, and produce, and on the other hand, they receive ignorance. In another idiom, we could say that humans are saved from bestiality through the gift of the imaginary and the symbolic order, but with this are given a dose of the Real and made to endure it as their lot.

Benardete permits us to appreciate the fundamental ambiguity of the gift because its repression of death throws out the baby with the bath since the awareness of mortality and death was part of the horizon of the sacred. So making death invisible also occurs at the cost of making the sacred invisible. This might be a poor exchange for humans because even without a sensitivity towards death and its oppressive aura, they must need something analogous to the sacred to handle the inevitable frustrations of life. The gift allows us to appreciate its impasse similar to the renowned Mafia offer of "your money or your life" or the offer we cannot refuse: here the gift of blindness offers us a life of inner peace, accept blindness to meaning or you shall be miserable, forlorn, and condemned to live with perpetual anxiety! Indeed, it seems as if a happy life requires the gift of blindness.

Here is the problem. If making death invisible (repressing it we would say) is a gift designed to remove the weight of anxiety over mortality and to enable humans to live at peace in time with the sense of purpose that life requires, this "gift" can still not eliminate anxiety because the life of knowledge (or the city as the Greeks said) is rife with expectation, aspiration, loss, dispossession, and all of the frustrations and aggressions to which we are heir, the overriding sense of longing and resentment, of the Oedipal imaginary that is correlative with life. The irony is that making death invisible actually makes tragedy and its pathos inevitable because we still need a way of handling anxiety.

The Law of the Symptom

Let us say that Prometheus guaranteed with his gift of repression that blindness would be our fate. This suggests that our life will be marked by the ways in which this plays out, how the blind adjust to their blindness and repression. Certainly if the return of the repressed is an ever-present part of our worldly horizon, our obituary might be read as a perpetual trajectory of defensive fortifications erected by the blind to protect against the return of the repressed. Is our fate to remain silent about death and to defend ourselves from the sight of death?

Walter Benjamin says that fate is misfortune elevated to the status of a law (1986, 304–311). The way this happens has been implicitly discussed in the literature as the work of symptom formation in Freud as the process through which a person defends herself from unwelcome thoughts through abreaction. Symptoms are adjustments developed over the course of a life to ward off unwelcome or "evil" thoughts that seem to us to jeopardize our security and sense of integrity and stability. It is as if one's mind cooperates with the body to ward off evil thoughts about oneself and the ambiguous border between the involuntary and voluntary character of such cooperation is continuously scrambled in evaluations of the subject by oneself or others. This suggests that the contingencies of a life become institutionalized in a deterministic formula. Fate designating this "law" supposedly belonging to the person is like a style imputed to the person as part of a characterization. This law that marks the person with an identifying stigma can make reference to what has been called the symptom. Symptoms are then both aesthetic and functional in Simmel's sense, as for example, when he discusses artifacts and objects such as the handle on a vase: if the symptom is functional by virtue of condensing and displacing some primordial anxiety, it is also aesthetic in the way it is composed as a kind of unified form, and has ethical implications that constrain and permeate all conduct. If in this way the symptom always appears to *be* the person, Benjamin cautions us not to treat such content as the character of the person because it is an adaptation to contingencies that have petrified into a formulaic style, almost a generic format, as a chance effect without purpose or design (as the character Timaeus says of such causes in the dialogue *Timaeus*) and not as if a result of oriented action towards ends "good and fair."

Benjamin's caution not to treat the symptom as character then leaves a space between our symptom as an apparent guise of who we are and our "real" self or the one we would want to be. Destiny then shows us that we must make something out of the symptom because life is not simply preparation for death but for the end as that destination where we work out what we accept as our fate and put such work into practice. In the idiom of the *Timaeus* our destiny is to relate with reason and intellect to the symptom that is our fate, to express a minded relation to the symptom. If we allow the symptom to rule us as if a law, we then accept its determination as if its content exhausts our character and as if our problem is to manage its volatility and its effects in order to maintain stability. More reflectively, we can always challenge our symptom and its infrastructure of defenses and try to expose its grounds as matters to take up and help clarify as possibilities for healing.

Fate describes how the element of causality enters thought as a force over time, occasioned by a traumatic apprehension of ambiguity that tends to disclose the working of mind as if a machine, apparently governed by its historical experiences in ways that are recurrent and seem to acquire the power of an inheritance both oppressive and yet open to modification. Thus, if conditions such as class, race, and gender seem as if external facts, it is mind itself and its causal powers that can make such conditions appear as if primary in contrast to the imagination that represents them as such. I use symptom in a similar sense to the usage developed by Didi-Huberman for his description of art history and its semiotic governance (Didi-Huberman 2005).

We can now begin to appreciate the world of tragedy as the world of a subject ruled by the chance and external force of the symptom because the symptom seems to personify what Timaeus calls "spurious causes" that "produces chance effects without order or design," which compel us to move but not towards that "which is fair and good" (see Plato's *Timaeus*, 1949). The world of tragedy seems to emphasize caring for and cultivating symptom management as its *sine qua non*. The problem of symptom management, that it cannot hold unruly jouissance at bay and channel it constructively, is confirmed by the anxieties of life that always "return" the repressed to its subject as matters to manage and to negotiate.

Parameters of Tragedy

The reversal of fortune that the canon identifies as a parameter of tragedy refers to the disruption of complacency. The reversal of fortune and descent of a person of high repute signify the eruption of anxiety in the world of tragedy when the tension between mortality and the lack of a poetic art to engage its limits is made unbearable. I suggest that these conventional parameters gloss the most fundamental disruption, which is the return of the repression of death, its reemergence in the world as the mark of the tragic consciousness.

Now we are forced to consider the tension between profane and sacred because we lost the illusion that we were total and complete rather than divided. Forgetting the tension of engaging this mix is due to the work of the symptom that masks it. The sacred shows us vividly that we are both finite and infinite, that we are a mix and not either/or one or the other, and that without the resources of a commitment to the Ought, we risk losing the poetic capacity to engage this mix as a vital and inconclusive conversation. Now we see that in giving us the gift of the repression of death and the expulsion of the sacred, Prometheus also gifted us with the symptom to use in our new world. The problem is that our repression of death is also repression of the sacred and so, though we forget death, we lack the sacred to fortify us in life. Repressing death cannot repress anxiety because life is correlative with anxiety and so when we ask, what can replace the sacred and what guise can this replacement take, we can only welcome the symptom and its surrogates for the support of the sacred it offers in images of absolutism whether with respect to self, other, doctrines, etc.

The symptom is the gift of self-deception, the result of Prometheus' infliction of blindness, and with it we also acquire the wherewithal of its playful and complex texture as a web to experimentally engage. Prometheus' error was to see death as the only cause of anxiety, forgetting the connection of life to evaluation through mediation of the Ought. But now we see that almost as a residue of the gift he left us with a little treasure chest of strategies and tactics for innovatively translating our engagement with the Ought into a ritualized landscape of seductive moments. Now we have to convert the vice of our blindness into a virtue, to make something of it. This poses the problem of how we might live through the world of tragedy since the sight of death threatens to intermittently return to diminish our blindness. Is this perhaps a way of reinstating Hannah Arendt's call to arms asking us to rethink the situation of her title essay in *Men in Dark Times*? (Arendt 1968)

Repression as Fetish: the Bourgeoisie

Freud allows us to engage the world of tragedy and the structure of repression that it seems to exhibit. That is, can we begin to examine the kinds of adjustments made to the invisibility of death? The Greeks first exhibited this in the city of

Oedipus. According to Benardete, we live by chance in such a world and if we turn to try to recover the sacred we risk experiencing the traumatic ground of the symptom. Our choices seem to be a vision of the intelligible foundation of life as terrifying ambiguity or letting things lie and living according to chance.

Bataille ([1973] 1989, 51), quite a different character than Gadamer, says in his idiomatic way that the ambiguity of the gift signifies to many betrayal, leading not only to hysteria and oppression but to depression and rage as well.

> The anxiousness to remain personally alive that establishes the person's individuality is linked to the integration of existence into the world of things … work and the fear of dying are interdependent … man is an individual to the extent that his apprehension ties him to the results of labor.

If death is forgotten as if a truth to be discarded, this gesture of forgetting can take many shapes, for example, discussed by Freud and Lacan as the repression that Gadamer mentions, or as disavowal that simply rejects the truth, or finally as foreclosure that ceases to speak about it as if its truth, conceded in a sense, is unspeakable. Bataille intimates that the first shape of repression lies in work, productivity, and what we might call the preoccupation of humans with worldly pursuits and things. As we suggested, this shape of forgetting death we can call *bourgeoisie*. That our being occupied by things means in its way that the disturbing character of death is displaced and channeled into some notion of our productivity that is designed to affirm our extension in some way, that our end is only apparent because we will continue to live in and through our labor and its effects. It has been noted that children are treated in such ways to affirm the fertility of unending heterosexuality.

The Sight of Death: Fascination/Return of the Repressed

We have a sequence of metaphors: the world of tragedy aka the world of dark times, of the return of the repressed, of post-traumatic stress. What repression represses is the desire to theorize as the fundamental poetic element in speech, representation, and action. In each case humans make adjustments to the ineffable and inscrutable poetic element in desire, which they have difficulty objectifying to and for their satisfaction, in each case trying to find a substitute object or scapegoat for their frustrations. The scapegoat, whatever its content, is typically a condition that is invested with the force of a primary cause rather than the real cause as if it is most responsible for the action (and in the case of deleterious action, functions as Wittgenstein said as an assignment of guilt). The sight of death is an arresting moment.

> Self containment—what Michael Fried would call absorption—is a state that Pouissin recognizes as simply and fully human...but also obviously, about what it is in human dealings with nature that *puts a stop to the present* and produces a fully human temporality—a discontinuity, a focus on the

> instantaneous as a specific event, a hushing and twisting and exteriorizing of the here and now. What is it that does this? What but the sight of death?
>
> (Clark 2006, 233–4)

Here is the rudimentary appearance of death for one aging: "I am still alive for Death and yet dead for Life. Now what life was left me? The boredom I had known before, solitude, my own company" (Pirandello 2005, 189)? Here is a more reflective character.

> He often thought about death but usually in pity for an animal or fish or seeing the dying grass in the fall or the monarch butterflies clinging to milkweed and feeding for the great funeral flight. Were they aware of it somehow, the strength it would take, the heroic strength? He thought about death, but he had never been able to imagine it, the unbeing while all else still existed. The idea of passing from this world to another, the next, was too fantastic to believe. Or that the soul would rise in a way unknown to join the infinite kingdom of God. There you would meet again all those you had once known as well as those you had never known, the countless dead in numbers increasing but never as great as the infinite. The only ones missing would be those who believed there was nothing afterwards, as his mother had said… . Whatever you believed would happen was what happened, Beatrice said. She would go to some beautiful place. Rochester she said as a joke.
>
> (Salter 2013, 289)

If the sight of death can produce tragedy in various ways correlative with its pathos, perhaps we can begin to resurrect the notion of fascination as a fixation upon its recurrent aura that we might think of as decadence. Plato's works suggest that the mix of mind and body that marks us is a constant source of fascination because its indeterminate and enigmatic character often challenges us to remake its constraints, conventions, and circumstances into something more vital in the way deadly conditions often inspire idealization as escape or defense. The *Timaeus*, in particular, suggests that the part we share with all things, our lowest common denominator, is both the unmanageable part of ourselves and as such, a continuous source of fascination. That our mixed nature is an unending source of fascination for us tells us something about ourselves, for the constraint of this mix tempts us to dramatize the apparent primacy of the part that limits us. Because the unmanageable part of ourselves discloses our limit, it works much like a secret that we try to conceal under the façade of self-control and self-determination. If disruption seems to produce tragedy, what can disrupt tragedy but the return of the repressed and the renewed fascination with death?

Now we ask: what can we learn about humans from this continuous and essential fascination with our unruliness? Could it be that dark times, post-traumatic stress, and the return of the repressed exercise a lure, a kind of appeal, by virtue of moving us to act, motivating us to make something out of the ungovernable, by inspiring us to perform at life? The fascination of temptation is reflected in our absorption by the question of how we might weather the storm, make something out of our conditions, find our voice, be inspired to see our relation to the condition as capable of intelligence.

In this very special sense the attraction of the lower order (for which Plato uses the body and its unruliness as a prop for irrationality and its omnipresence in the soul) and the basis of its appeal lies in the fact that it *is* alien, mute and indifferent to value, and that its absence of meaning says that it must be given life. This attraction, often called decadence, is inspired by the imperative of giving life to the lowly, by the opportunity to breathe life into the dead. The project of rising to the occasion by managing the unmanageable (including meaninglessness) is the basis for developing an art of life, for performing or working-through instead of merely repeating under the spell of conditions. In this sense it is the very absence of meaning in any condition, which is conveyed in the mute signifier, word, image, that always needs to be invested with life that makes possible imaginative action. This is to say that life needs the otherness of death to be itself, leading us to appreciate how in a world without death life would have no weight for there would be nothing other to it and it could only be vacuous and formless. This is how Simmel can say that death has "form-giving significance" for life. I suggest that it is because such a sight inspires us not simply to continue exercising ourselves in practicing at life or to duplicate its expectations but to work it through in a way that invests it with the spirit of passion for performing and recharging its script.

In discussing theatrical practice in dramatic acting, the Israeli philosopher and actor Tzachi Zamir distinguishes the commitment to repetition in acting from mere exercise and duplication as two other shapes of mimetic action (Zamir 2010, 209). True repetition, he says, does not simply maintain or duplicate the normative but invests it with an affective tone by embodying its resonances in ways that make manifest inflections it can only hold in abeyance. This is akin to Freud's notion of *durcharbeiten* as working-through. Fascination with the lower order is a dedicated concern for the inspirational promise that the impersonal condition offers in its very indifference and silence. As Simmel also has said, true repetition in dramatic action invests the script (the alien condition, the text of life) with spirit. Here, I am equating what Zamir calls true repetition or performance with theorizing that works-through the representation and invests it with meaning by empowering the relationship that it assumes.

The complexity of the notion of decadence is now transparent in the ambiguity of such absorption, making intelligible the conception of fascination itself, on the one hand reveling in the degradation of the lowly—the orthodoxa, inert signifier, the cliché—and on the other, as being moved by the challenge of the mute condition (its conventionality, its being a word and nothing more), to breathe life into it by seeing it as a giving of the gift of life that invites us to test and confirm *our* vitality in bringing it to life. The condition—naked and open-ended—always tests our creativity: do we resign ourselves to it, treating it as self-evident, or do we desire to try to make something more of it? The arts of painting, dance, cinema, writing, all begin with images sanctified in clichés that reflect the mechanization of relationships to what might be seen, heard, spoken, touched, and in the best of cases from such beginnings can charge such images with meaning and life. If, as Hegel says, habit is the mechanization of self-feeling, true repetition always invests habit with life, measuring itself by finding its voice through its embodiment of habit in the action of performance. Zamir lets us see that a world without death is a world that has lost its gift for performance insofar as action that performs at life first needs its absorption in the mute condition in order to take flight and to escape from its habituated character, its chance or randomness in order to give the condition value (in the language of Plato, to be erotic). A world without death is a world imagined as without figurative language. A world without death, without performance and its artifice, without the as-if and without illusion, seems the horizon of the world of tragedy and the governance of symptom management. We might now make better sense of Aristotle's notion of comedy as the imitation of low life. Perhaps this begins to connect the enigmatic smile of the Mona Lisa to the Pygmalion fantasy and Baudelaire's idealization of the woman as the icon of artistic pursuit, all disclosing in their very different ways the capacity of silence to fertilize creativity as recognized from the sages through Lacan's affirmation that Other does not answer. That we need the deadly reminder that Prometheus repressed in order to correct or at least supplement our blindness is certainly worth a laugh.

This is the turning point for the movement to comedy, the recognition that we are dealing with figures of speech for the relationship within each of us between a lower and higher part, indications of the varying moments of a stream of consciousness interior and internal in which we double ourselves, seeing our unity as a two-in-one, where higher and lower parts inevitably and perennially collide in ways that might always give pause, often appearing pathetic, ludicrous, and comedic because the persistent attempt to master the stream is both necessary, desirable, and impossible to fulfill, animated by a dream of phallic consummation that is still only foreplay. This is to say something that has not been said before: comedy is the gesture that laughs at what it must try, specifically the desire to make foreplay consummation. Is this not a way to relate to Kenneth Burke's comment on making a virtue out of our vice, or Lacan's conception of converting our symptom into a sinthome? For example, in the best of comedy, what Baudelaire calls "absolute humor" (1972), the subject is induced to recognize its automated relation to externalized customs that it has made certain and unconditional without reflection, for example, the inevitability of death and the fantasies of loss that it encourages. The subject of absolute humor knows that life is both foreplay and to be treated with sexual finality, needing and desiring to perform at life as if it knows not of death while knowing full well that it does.

Here, the relationship to life is oriented to the recognition that its mix makes its lower order *seem* primary. Thus, the comic thrust of all art is meant to reveal not merely the empirical limits of norms (death *will* happen and so will the losses it imagines) but the need and desire to represent the drive of life and its infinite perplexity as necessary and absolute rather than contingent, the need to represent customs such as the self as equipment for living, as matter both automated and malleable, made over recurrently in the way that laughing at this remains a matter of life and death. What this suggests is that the project(s) that prevents our engagement with mortality through the repression it stimulates is redesigned in the drive to live. If melancholy seems true in its way, this truth might be false in relation to the Real, false in relation to the as-if of the drive of life and its artifice, raising the perennial questions what is true and what is its relationship to the Real?

Life as an Aesthetic Phenomenon

If death is treated as a condition that limits us from thinking poetically or as a constraint upon us that neutralizes the desire we conceive as aesthetic, then we begin to appreciate the two-sidedness driving the division of the subject and its development as a relationship to language that enables us to begin to give form to material conditions in ways that give form to theorizing as an uncanny embodiment, as both escape and sacrificial, and so, as driven in its relentlessness, in its very jouissance that is the death drive revealed in Socratic ignorance (that the truth has to be pursued even and in so far as we know that we do not know). This is to say that an aesthetic relation to the "original division" of the subject makes reference to an ideal speaker able to double herself as two-in-one ("in other words, the identity of a subject capable of escaping the assignment to a private condition and of intervening in the affairs of the community") (Rancière, 2009, 6). Here, the "affairs of the community" could be the common language, its *doxa* and familiar distinctions and proper names ("that pin people down") and the "escape" from the private assignment can be not simply rejection but what Rancière calls ("a transgressive affirmation") a reformulation aiming to reassign meaning to what had been privately assigned, the second sailing, where what had been thought is rethought as if for the second time. Because it is a social order (the symbolic order) that "assigns" us to a private condition and its name, that assignment includes for any one so subject, a capacity for "escape." This escape begins to make reference to the powers of disengagement that we might call aesthetic, a capacity to seem to be at home with what is temporary and contingent and at the same time to be desirous of something other, to be two in one as reflected in the division or ban honored in the lingo of Lacan. This capacity for escape is included in the symbolic order itself as the hole in Being (Lacan) or desire that is necessary and exempt, a necessary exemption, an exemption both necessary and desirable, that comes to view for an aesthetic eye.

If the notion of Grey Zone seems to point to the omnipresence of ambiguity as loss or a "fall" from some definitive standard of exactitude, or even as a lack or deficiency accompanying the so-called alienation of modern society, the strong conception of ambiguity can only understand it as appearing in different shapes that occlude not perfect clarity but an elemental notion of ambiguity itself that is intrinsic to the human being as (in the words of Plato) both original and image, as the constant and ever-present passage between these registers.

> The difficulty, henceforth, to look at what remains (visible) while summoning up what had disappeared; in short, to scrutinize the visual traces of this

> disappearance, which I will otherwise call (and without any clinical connotations): its symptoms.
>
> (Didi-Huberman 2005, 50)

The development of life as the repressed story of the relationship integral to any image (say, the destiny of the one who dies, who has died, who must and will die), is not a task of looking backward to fill in hermeneutic detail for what has been eclipsed, or to look ahead for guarantees, but to enjoy performing at whatever might, through its eloquence, rescue the image from the oblivion of repression. In the way that such a death drive brings to life an object (the representation of the canon itself not as "great books" or aesthetic objects nor as ruling discriminations but as an influence brought to life as in the gesture of *prosopopeia)*, the death drive seems life's version of its existence as art, of the art of life not as art history or museology but as the aesthetic justification noted by Nietzsche, to perform at life in the shadow of death, the desire to enact hyperbolically the action that can renounce the temptation of inaction as if unaware, suffering the mix of pleasure and pain that such a pose must inherit.

That is, to apprehend death aesthetically is not to see it in terms of its causal structure, material composition, nor as desirable or not, for these conditions that apply to the social representation of death do not evoke its intimate singularity, its "who" rather than what. To say that "aesthetic apprehension of a form is without concept" (Rancière 2009) echoes Simmel's injunction to provide form to material conditions, to rethink the phenomenon not in terms of its efficiency or desirability, but as a representation accompanied by a certain ignorance (that is, knowledge of one's limits or in Lacan, of the hole in the symbolic order as a modernization of the maxim of Socratic ignorance). In this way, Rancière after Lacan and others finds oppressiveness not in death *per se* but in these ways of representing death (as knowledge, as undesirable) that neutralize an aesthetic relationship to speech.

> It is thus that such experience is much more than appreciating works of art. It concerns the definition of a type of experience which neutralizes the circular relationship of knowledge as know-how and knowledge as the distribution of roles. Aesthetic experience eludes the sensible distribution of roles and competences which structures the hierarchical order.
>
> (Rancière 2009, 4)

Conclusion

Comedy and tragedy are typically treated as interlocutors but Baudelaire's distinction between ordinary and absolute humor suggests that the notion of humor can be seen as a problem-solving situation that sets into play the difference between these types of comedic engagements within humor itself as its two parts rather than between comedy and whatever is outside of it and that "real" comedy develops as a way of making manifest that distinction. Baudelaire then invites us to focus upon the form of comedy before trying to connect it to externals. Let us say that the tragic view of life makes possible, palatable, and comforting one conception of comedy as ordinary humor in and through its very pathos, and also offers resources for developing the absolute humor that Baudelaire identifies as true to the spirit of comedy. Whereas ordinary humor builds on the Oedipal imaginary and its typical effects of longing, resignation, dispossession, frustration, and aggression, absolute humor tries to overcome such a limit by performing in ways that could look the same and/or different. A strong version of comedy depends upon formulating a subject orienting to a self-reflective vision of the self as split, experienced as both intimate, singular and feeling, and as objectified in the way of a thing, thrown into life as both, as mixed, what Mario Perniola calls a thing that feels or a feeling thing, given such title in life in many ways and constructed as needing and desiring to improvise under external conditions by sending up one's own alien and objectified appearance in performing imaginative resolutions. Such performing takes shape in tactile relationships to language that celebrate its ambiguity as an enjoyable and hyperbolic relation to convention that is inherited by the self as if an order both alien and malleable. Such an actor, in the idiom of Baudelaire, both dual and acting as if unaware of this duality, necessarily takes up the figures of the fool as we said, or the clown, the puppet as one who acts as if master of their fate while knowing full well that they are subject to the weight of this as-if. This makes comedy appear both grave and amused, always deadly serious in its clowning around with language and action.

References

Aeschylus. 1956. "Prometheus Bound." In *Aeschylus II: The Complete Greek Tragedies.* Edited by David Grene and Richmond Lattimore. New York: Washington Square Press.

Améry, Jean. 1994. *On Aging: Revolt and Resignation.* Translated by John Barlow. Bloomington and Indianapolis: Indiana University Press.

Arendt, Hannah. 1968. *Men in Dark Times.* New York: Harcourt Brace and Company.

Bataille, Georges. (1973) 1989. *Theory of Religion.* Translated by Robert Hurley. New York: Zone Books.

Baudelaire, Charles. 1972. "On the Essence of Laughter, and Generally of the Comic in the Plastic Arts." In *Selected Writings on Art and Artists*, translated by P.E. Charvet, 140–61. Harmondsworth: Penguin.

Baudrillard, Jean. 1987. *The Evil Demon of Images.* Sydney: Robert Burton.

Benjamin, Walter. 1986. "Fate and Character." In *Reflections.* Edited by Peter Demetz, translated by Edmund Jephcott. New York: Schocken.

Benardete, Seth. 2000. "On Greek Tragedy." In *The Argument of the Action: Essays on Greek Poetry and Philosophy*, 99–145. Chicago: University of Chicago Press.

Blum, Alan. 2011. *The Grey Zone of Health and Illness.* Bristol: Intellect Press.

Clark, T.J. 2006. *The Sight of Death: An Experiment in Art Writing.* New Haven and London: Yale University Press.

DeLeuze, Gilles and Felix Guattari. (1980) 1987. *A Thousand Plateaus: Capitalism and Schizophrenia.* Translated by Brian Massumi. Minneapolis: University of Minnesota Press.

Didi-Huberman, Georges. (1990) 2005. *Confronting Images.* University Park PA: The Pennsylvania State University Press.

Gadamer, Hans-Georg. (1993) 1996. *The Enigma of Health: The Art of Healing in a Scientific Age*. Translated by John Gaiger and Nicholas Walker. Stanford: Stanford University Press.

Garfinkel, Harold, 1967. *Studies in Ethnomethodology.* Englewood Heights, NJ: Prentice Hall.

Hesiod. 1953. *Theogony*. Indianapolis and New York: Bobbs-Merrill.

Negrete, Fernanda. 2015. "'A Vital, Unliveable Force:' Rhythm Through Nathalie Sarraute and Schizoanalysis." *Mosaic* 48 (2): 83–98.

Nietzsche, Friedrich. 1956. *The Birth of Tragedy and the Geneaology of Morals.* Translated by F. Golffing. New York: Doubleday.

Perniola, Mario. (2000) 2004. *The Sex Appeal of the Inorganic: Philosophies of Desire in the Modern World.* Translated by Massimo Verdicchio. New York and London: Continuum.

Pirandello, Luigi. 2005. *The Late Mattia Pascal.* Translated by William Weaver. New York: New York Review of Books.

Plato. 1949. *Timaeus*. Translated by B. Jowett. Indianapolis: Library of the Liberal Arts.

Rancière, Jacques. 2009. *Aesthetics and its Discontents.* Walden, MA: Polity Press.

Salter, James. 2013. *All That Is.* New York: Alfred A. Knopf.

Sarraute, Nathalie. 1963. *The Age of Suspicion.* Translated by Maria Jolas. New York: George Brailler.

Wallace, David Foster. 1988. Afterword to *Wittgenstein's Mistress*, by David Markson. Champaign, Dublin, London: Dalkey Archive Press.

Zamir, Tzachi. 2009. "Theatrical Repetition and Inspired Performance." *Journal of Aesthetics and Art Criticism* 67 (4): 365–373.

——. 2010. "Puppets." *Critical Inquiry* 36 (3): 386–419.

—— 2010. "Watching Actors." *Theatre Journal* 62 (2): 227–243.

12 The Travesty of End-of-Life

Introduction

I started this book by positing an impasse that I explored through the narrative and that I must return to as its irresolute conclusion. I began by restating the enigmatic query from Sophocles' chorus on whether not to be born might be the greatest boon of all. I dramatized this query as if a proposition intending to provoke reflection on the life of the dying body. Non-being as this sense of being unborn seems impossible to imagine and this possibility of impossibility accounts in part for our fear of death. Yet, the Greeks believed that acute suffering could cause us to reach for such an impossible image and in desperate circumstances to try to imagine it as a choice we might have. Indeed, could life cause us to choose being unborn as preferable to what it has to offer? Yet as we said at the outset, life seems impossible to reject in most cases though our acceptance is not simply habitual but tinged with anxiety. Here we begin to appreciate the figures of escape and flight in everyday life and its imaginative infrastructure. My use of this enigmatic refrain of the Greek chorus is a gesture designed to unsettle our relationships to life as part of social inquiry into our imaginative structure. The fragility of such a structure can be expected to become most visible at the end-of-life and it is the situation of aging in our society that I will briefly address at this point.

The Phenomenology of the Present

At any time the wide-awake aged subject knows that absorption in the current environment is both necessary and desirable (for progress, enhancing humane values, and perhaps for their own integrity as being up-to-date and involved in the lives of their contemporaries and/or intimates or as dissociated and disengaged), but as such, seems to require a mode of concentration that, in the words of Rilke, is once and no more. Such an awareness can create a distance towards the present and its activities and this temptation has the force to compromise the involvement of the aged in their environment and by virtue of this, in the activities of those around them. Whether apparent or real, the experience of this temptation remains a condition to be oriented to by both the elderly and the relevant others in their environments to mark aging as a case of mutually oriented social action (Weber

1947). We have spoken of togetherness and apartness, and boundary ambiguity as figures of speech for this mixed relation to the present moment that needs to be displayed, whether mobilized or feigned, as a sign of the participation of the aged at any present moment. The aged social actor knows that every present seems to swamp its subject with an array of incidental activities and courses of action that demand urgent concentration and attention, which at the same moment still promise to fade and become at best upon future review a past memory and nothing more. Yet, the aged know that they must act as if this present moment is eternal while knowing that it will perish. The problematic figure of the aged subject in relation to commitment to the present is a crucial feature of this social situation. Thus, the ideal subject of end-of-life might be guided by Baudelaire's maxim for absolute humor in the knowledge that we act with vigor in our commitment to the present while being aware of the relativism of this gesture.

In this way the duality of Baudelaire's comic relationship and its two minds in one comes alive as the unawareness feigned in action knowing better. To conceive of a way of life under the auspices of the subject in this manner as the course of action that this figure recommends, that is, to live knowing this, to live in the manner of such a subject, invites us to rethink death as a relationship embodied in practice, in oriented action that we can reveal as the way(s) the relationship to death is to be lived and suffered. Of course, end-of-life gives us an opportunity to observe this scene. In other words, if death appears both relative and absolute in senses we have discussed, such a relationship needs to be embodied as such, as that disengagement from the fatality of condition and content that could permit any of us to move freely, perhaps bringing to mind the figure of the aesthetic relationship through Simmel's metaphor of the stranger as one who comes and goes, is here today and gone tomorrow. The view of such a present can be inspiring when linked to particular circumstances through the opportunities they present for analysis, opportunities as data that are invariably accidental and yet elicited in ways that provide occasions for playfully making passing time significant.

Death Drive

The jouissance of the death drive, beyond the pleasure principle insofar as it mixes both pleasure and pain, is captured by Simmel and particularly in his portrait of Casanova who desired the impossible.

> To the sober person adventurous conduct often seems insanity; for, in order to make sense, it appears to presuppose that the unknowable is known.
>
> (Simmel 1971, 194)

The problem of the death drive (following from the finitude of *dasein,* the human being) and from its division or duality—is that it needs and desires to do the impossible, for example, to achieve complete clarification, even in the face of its knowledge that it is partial (divided). The lived experience of the dying body must relinquish both fixation upon death and detachment towards death—both views at once—by determining to be determinate in performing at life in its present, knowing that in doing that and that alone, it sacrifices knowledge for ignorance while doing ignorance in a way meant to embody knowing this and only this. That is, in acting as if we are ignorant while knowing that we are not—in acting as if we are eternal while knowing our destination is death—we remain ruled by both our absolutistic faith in our eternality and our relativistic sense of our shared mortality, both at once, divided as such.

If on the one hand we are not superior to nature but simply another part of life, a thing that thinks (Perniola 2004), ruled by the fateful inheritance of our symptom, our thinking still purports to elevate us, to maintain an apartness by virtue of this mere trifle. That we have this and this alone, togetherness and apartness, is the story we desire to represent in word, deed, and through our influences, the story as our necessary dream, our equipment for living.

At one and the same time, the momentum of this narrative sustains the division in its own practice between our commitment to the common view that leads us to act as if our life is eternal in the face of the shadow of death *and* our detachment that exaggerates the sense of a problem that animates this view to which we *seem* compliant, showing our being gripped by the perennial and vexatious temptation of reflection when we are touched by the grace of imagination—am I part of society or apart? The pleasure of sexual finality resides in its nerve to say "both!" with the force of exaggeration designed to excite both those who think they are apart from society and not a part (the robotic rejection of death), and those who think that they are only a part of society and could never defend being apart (the automated rejection of life because of the inevitability of death). For us, the spectacle of working through this lived experience of death is most vivid typically at the end-of-life when it seems for the wide-awake (and even Heraclitus' sleepwalkers) that it is most difficult to avoid the question.

Life as Travesty

Since the lived experience of the dying body typically might be understood to expire the closer we get to the end-of-life, old age can be expected to mirror in an exemplary and dramatic manner the anxieties surrounding this engagement. In the previous chapters, I have tried to develop a path towards a reflective relationship to death, not wishfully but in terms of action, and it is important to try to think through the embodiment of a relationship to death in the life of the aged as a possible demonstration of the tension of such a reflective engagement and perhaps the prospect for a degree of healing. Even the euphemistic refrain that speaks of aging as maturity and of the empowered position that seems to make possible the potential for an elderly overview of history and life is difficult to see as anything more than a lament. Within such a context, the problem always appears to be one of adapting to the loss or disadvantage that end-of-life brings and this aura of loss is of course signaled by the proximity of impending death.

In this book, I have travestied the spellbound hold of life on us by trying to examine the force of the aura of non-being in everyday life. This is the impasse I begin with and can only resolve plaintively. In the last chapter, I identified a comedic relation to mortality as our "equipment for living," our "best practices," but this remains abstract until we can begin to observe the practice(s) of such courses of action in life. The strong relation to death that I have tried to imagine, materializing in my vision of a reflective engagement with mortality, should be observable selectively as a potential intrinsic in the practices at the end-of-life in the shape of an impasse revealing possibilities that can be taken up or not, that are both definitive and open-ended. Can we use the end-of-life as an opportunity to observe aging as the paradigmatic example of Baudelaire's comedic relationship to mortality since the immanence of a mortal end seems most vivid then to even the sluggish? What kind of engagement would this look like as it would certainly be instructive for anyone and everyone? That is, such a possibility for the lived experience of the dying body might be imagined if we could test it by observing such possible practices at end-of-life.

Aging in Modern Life

If many emphasize how modern society orients to change and its mastery as a guiding expectation, we have to consider what particular pressures this concern imposes upon the experience of aging. As I developed the idea from Guy Swanson's work (Blum 2003, 56–59), the orientation to change is a sign of modernization and applicable to every social phenomenon (Swanson 1971, 138–9). That is, in line with the modern evaluation of change as necessary and desirable, people too are expected to change and to adapt to evolving circumstances in ways that can only put the idea of inheritance and history under pressure. When such an emphasis is made to include categories such as the aged, obsolescence and contemporaneity are always grounds for characterizing modes of adjustment.

The categories of time and space are instructive here, for not only societies change, but the figure of time reveals how such change is registered in the modification of old ways that can invariably frustrate the subject, while the figure of space discloses the force of migration where old lives are exchanged for new ones and disappearance and relearning become preoccupations of subjects on the move (Blum 2003, 88–114). Here the connection of globalization to aging invariably presents the elderly with such challenges of situating themselves in relation to acquiring new methods, and making the problem of adaptation a perennial project for the elderly who reside in one changing place over time and/or who migrate from their places to new situations.

Concretely, in terms of time, in any one society the elderly risk being out of step unless they adapt, and in relation to space, as newcomers the old seem always out of step unless they relearn, making adaptation as a task not only everyone's problem, but a problem that takes particular shape for the elderly. Since the commitment to change assumes a relation to the future in the present and an openness to the possibility of influencing the future, the particular situation of the aged is invariably connected to their belief in what lies ahead. What I have suggested throughout is that this optimism is shadowed by the sense of the inevitability of death that must require an almost hallucinatory drive to bracket or suspend. Further, in the absence of any universal standard for adjustment, the demand to adapt must take its bearings from the conventions and normative order of the place into which the elderly are "thrown," the social standards or "generalized other" of such a place of settlement. Within such a context, the sensitive among the aged can always be wary and cautious towards the unreflective enthusiasms of any present. This reserve tends to elicit animosity in return towards the elderly who appear reluctant to accept such enthusiasms as eo ipso "interesting," always creating reciprocal propensities for either acting out or for the concealment of feelings. Thus, short of abuse, the elderly are often typified in terms of three kinds of characterizations that can be converted into accusations: first, for their idleness as when they are told to "get a life;" secondly, because of such supposed idleness, as failing to perform according to routine expectations such as assisting with domestic chores in serving the nuclear family; and finally, as burdensome interruptions of family who expect them to persevere, if lucky, with their own kind in sites for assisted living because they are assumed to enjoy being with those who seem to be similar because of their age. Reciprocally, the elderly retaliate against their once intimate relationships for lack of loyalty and gratitude as part of an imaginary of indebtedness that pervades this discourse.

Within such a context the preoccupation with what is called "successful aging" confirms the recognition that aging remains an unhappy attempt to adapt to circumstances that seem to offer no advantage, with "success" disclosing how the special character of such a group remains its need to overcome a situation that has deteriorated for them, a problem of surviving or regaining not what was lost but self-composure in a situation of loss. Success is defined either as conforming pacifically to local standards and/or trying to maintain an interest in being productive in ways legitimized by these standards (Baltes and Baltes 1990; Dillaway 2009). We shall return to this notion of successful aging as the good adaptation shortly.

The Problem of Aging

One problem that aging raises immediately concerns the question of what kind of loss it appears to be since growing old is invariably identified as a loss (in popular culture, of bodily capacities, of security of employment or income, perhaps of respect, or of self-confidence). Aging is not seen as an advantage, though the character of Cephalus in Plato's Republic claims that he is happy to be free of the bondage of eros as if that is the distracting force of sexuality, or of the so called eros that is supposed to saturate ambition, work, and productivity, which is a typical rhapsody of the aged in relation to retirement as if they are then free to be creative in their uses of time unshackled by their oppressive working routines. As I showed (Blum 2011), Socrates revealed this satisfaction to be linked to Cephalus' wealth that made his aging more comfortable and Socrates also implied that it was a one-sided view. As I have proposed in this work, eros properly understood is a necessary resource of the aged when it is appreciated as the ground of a poetic engagement with the life of the present in any period. Moreover, research suggests that even when all of the support is in place there is great anxiety, for example money is not enough for the vulnerable elderly treated mechanically or dutifully in their families or settings, just as social relationships provide company but often not autonomy or intimacy. Here, even if the elderly report that they are satisfied or tell themselves this, a darkness typically remains, the "foreign intruder" we discovered throughout.

The question of the loss must refer to deeper concerns than the alleviation or not of these transient conditions: If the problem of end-of-life is one of dealing with loss, what is reputed to be lost with growing years is some sense of the prime of life or some self-understanding of one's expectations regarding influencing the future. If we suggest that what is lost is that sense of optimism, what is meant as a loss is a firm orientation to temporality or to one's existence in time.

Eros of Aging

The relation to time becomes dramatic when the realization "strikes" that the future is out of our control, and our past, so singular and memorable, will perish with us in ways that can leave only uncertainty. In this sense, the problem of living only in a present, knowing the present is all there is, can invite the desperation or at best resignation we have discussed throughout or the commitment to the present as an arena for more than doing time, an opportunity to perform at life here and now knowing full well the necessity of such an hallucination. Eros then becomes relevant as this desire to renew our life at this time and in this way. Note, according to a journalist, how the writer Stefan Zweig expressed this when he treated even his impending fiftieth year as a crisis in a letter to his wife at the height of his productivity and repute:

> " ... a crisis growing out of advancing years, tied up with uncompromising clarity of insight ... I am not fooling myself with dreams of immortality, know how relative all literature is, don't have any faith in mankind, derive enjoyment from too few things... . I expect nothing from the future; it's a matter of indifference to me whether I sell 10,000 or 150,000 copies. The important thing would be to make a new beginning with something new, a different way of life, to have different ambitions, to have a different relationship to being, to emigrate but not merely in the physical sense of the word." Two years later he wrote: "I feel as if the screws are coming loose in the machine: the best thing would be to switch it off completely in its fiftieth year and make another attempt to experience the world again instead of describing it"
>
> (Zweig 2012, ix–x).

For this writer the only alternative path out of despair over the abyss of an eternal present is to erotically seize the moment by imagining a new life, a new way into being in the present almost as if remaking oneself. This marks desire as more than sexual but as libidinal at its best, reveling in its performing in a new way, the opportunity to fantasize its consequentiality while knowing full well the limits. In this way this connection I have made throughout to Baudelaire's absolute humor is the theoretic template for Zupančič's contrast of weak and strong versions of comedy in which this engagement imitates the excess of life (Zupančič 2008) by playing at the logos as if becoming the universal, the joke and not the joker, the illustrated and not the illustrator. If the project animating the reflective aged subject in any present is to recover and revitalize an innocence that is lost, the risk is always the appearance of childishness and frivolity.

Aging and Change

Renewing oneself in the present raises the question of whether the elderly, steadfast and supposedly tied to inheritances that are fixed and unyielding, can break away in any present to put new touches on what is being passed on. The writer Zweig speaks of such change as a necessity but as a dream that is problematic. The question: "can the aging subject change?" always appears to ask if the aging can adapt to changing circumstances by living under their rule, conforming to the regime of their present in terms of which they might seem obsolete. Zweig implies that real change must be more than adapting to circumstances, such as accepting retirement, going to the residence for "assisted living," inhabiting as a dependent and grateful presence the domicile of family and relatives, because these are all adjustments to changing conditions that affect the elderly but is not the kind of change that Zweig mentions in "experiencing the world" anew or in "migrating' intellectually and imaginatively. His question asks whether or not the aging subject can remake oneself in new ways, can perform at an art of life, or must only accept the altered circumstances as conventions that compel adaptation? If the aging are comparable to Zweig and fortunate enough to have his "uncompromising clarity of insight" (those for whom this book is written) then the question always remains: how can the elderly live or what kind of life can they be expected to pursue? There is no algorithmic answer here though many researchers have tried to define for the others (those for whom I am not writing) a convention called "successful aging" that is intended to give satisfaction to many responsible for aging friends and relatives or for one's own peace of mind in this difficult period. Indeed, one question this book asks in terms of the impasse is whether it might be better not to be born than to have such "uncompromising clarity of insight?"

The Panic Discourse: Aging and Materialism

Interlocutors to this "uncompromising clarity of insight" that the writer Zweig reflects are many, typical, and representative of the normal and conventional view(s) of our modern society towards the phenomenon of aging. That these views are necessary for putting the depressing thought of death to rest in any present shows the impasse in any commitment to the present almost as if we must settle on ignorance itself as our virtue, as equipment for living. In fact, is it not this "suspension" of any concern for meaning that makes the celebration of behaviorism in all of its forms alive and well, apparently intelligible and "rational" as in "big data" fetishism and the dedication to neurological resolutions of quandaries? For example, is it not better to be dead (in relation to meaning) than beset with the problems and anxieties that irresolution, ambiguity, and the concern for meaning release?

In this sense one factor that aging reveals quite dramatically is the way the celebration of life frequently voiced by the elderly is an affirmation of survival itself in the way gratitude for being alive must exclude any concern with quality of the life survived. In this way the limited case of surviving desperate circumstances can be used to enable survivors to evaluate the life they maintain as good simply by virtue of surviving it. This desperation model of survival haunts the discourse at many levels: the migrant who arrives in a country, any country, finds it a good place simply because they have arrived, as if the question of the quality of the place is irrelevant. In the same way, the incumbent of a job in a market situation with high unemployment and job scarcity is fortunate to have a position under such circumstances without respect to the quality of the job. Here again we see the interlocutor to the refrain of the Greek chorus that it is better not to be born, in this affirmation of the panic discourse that we're lucky to be alive and that it is a sin to be depressed, almost subversive to be reflective in that way (see Chapter 5 of this volume).

The Complex Presence of the Elderly

The emphasis on change characteristic of modern life marks the aged as particularly vulnerable as a target for indictment. This is due to the power of the belief in the relevance of the present for the future and of the human capacity to be productive, the commitment to the present as an opportunity and to the future as a probable realization of such present opportunism and dedication. The elderly seem, when conspicuous in their withdrawal, to resist the relationship to productivity, capable of making transparent the illusion itself.

That is, the limits of the emphasis on productivity which are ever-present but masked by an absorption in worldly activities, can only come to view in the visible suffering of end-of-life as an apparent terminal condition, much like the climax of a chronic disease. Unless the aged are inclined to accept gracefully this period as defined only by the external condition such as illness, financial hardship, unemployment, and the like, they invariably risk appearing as a ghostly reminder of what Bataille has called the betrayal of life. In this way the aged are always a complex presence in the midst of a productive society, capable of exposing the grounds of social life in the hallucination that its intimate and co-creative synergy will continue as it is forever.

In an interesting inversion then, if we follow Goffman's model of cooling the mark out that stresses how the more advantaged provide consolation in order to pacify the resentment of those who have suffered in any way and particularly at their hands (Goffman 1952). We might suggest as an alternative that it is not as typically thought to be "society" that cools out its elderly (though all social policy definitely has this inflection), but is the aged (when reflective) who must understand their task in any present as one of cooling out the society (friends, intimates, associates) and to distract them from confronting their limits without mediation.

This two-sided separation of end-of-life, either as a stage of "normal" decline or a sign of intransigence, helps organize relationships of care and treatment of the aged: in care it is advantageous to see the orientation of the elderly whatever its quality, less as an expression of dissatisfaction, and if seeming to be unhappy, to be caused by external conditions rather than by the unsettling and aporetic question of the meaning and point of their lives and of life per se. The policies of caregiving, when guided by surveys of elderly preferences and so-called "happiness," must miss the point that false consciousness or agreeableness can only conceal the fundamental anxiety of end-of-life as a concern that inventories of attitudes can never touch. The inability of the aged and the others to speak together, no matter how good-hearted, testifies to the fundamental otherness of the relationship: on the one hand, revealing a difference greater than those signified by classifications such as gender, race, or class because it is a difference between those who have and have not a sense of future (though extreme cases of social class and opportunity structure resonate in a related way), and on the other hand, an inability to treat (for the reflective) those who are similar as anything more than incumbents of a category. That the elderly are expected to enjoy the company of those categorized as similar—imagine the so-called peer group of 80 year olds who delight in being together by virtue of being the same age—can only dramatize the way such a category must always exclude its variations or otherness, disclosing how the aged and the others cannot speak to one another except under the façade of shared commitment to a future and how the aged cannot speak to one another except under the façade of a shared commitment to being at the same period of life. What Max Weber diagnosed as the inner isolation of the subject of capitalism is dramatized in the figure of the impasse of solitude at end-of-life, the pathos of those straining to be creative if possible, and typically compliant and resigned in relation to those who cannot or will not yet find such a destination intelligible.

How then can the aged navigate this tension between the morbid resignation of the reflective writer and the fragile compliance of those who must put the thought of death to rest in their fantasies of retirement, assisted living, and domestic sanctuary? Is there a path for a reflective relationship to life (and not only for the aged) that can begin to operate between the extremes of suicidal despair and ignorance to solve the problem of administering jouissance in the present, in any present?

The Destination of End-of-Life: Sisyphus, Zombie, Clown

If Sisyphus epitomizes futility, seeming to do what is required on the surface (perhaps those "normal" aged who do elderly recreation pursuits in whatever context, appearing alive but perhaps dead inside), when we encounter the forlorn and aged on our streets who live in extreme circumstances of deprivation, they seem as if zombies. The zombie then accentuates and brings to view the malaise concealed in the movement of Sisyphus. We need to imagine alternatives that can help us position ourselves positively in relation to the enigmatic refrain of the Greek chorus—an alternative to Sisyphus and the Zombie—in order to begin to formulate a stronger relationship to the end-of-life for all concerned.

Recall Freud's affirmation of love as a power that conquers death: if this sounds like narcissism there still might be a way to acknowledge self-love as something other than limited egoism but as the love for oneself as respect for one's capacity to exemplify more than a contingent relation to conditions, a commitment to the desire to enhance desire (for more than life), the desire to perform as if engaging a new life in the writer Zweig's sense, perhaps the desire to regain that kind of innocence. Self-love could then be seen as the desire for desire in the sense of desiring something more of oneself, a capacity to motivate oneself to rise above a conditional existence not by exceeding others in productivity but by exemplifying some strong sense of what it is to be human. To love humanity might be to desire to preserve its inborn excess as including the way such eros must mark the two sides of its desire for life and for more than life, and the impasse of living through and in the contradiction of being in-between that this impasse imposes as an inheritance.

Both Plato and Freud converge in recognizing this procreative component of eros, this desire to overstep boundaries and to perform at being more than a scarecrow of determinism in Benjamin's sense. In this book I have used inquiry and art as a conjunctive image of such desire for self-transcendence, tempered by absolute humor, as the image of a path that preserves its mix as absolute and relative. Yet, more seems to me to be needed to save this book from ending as a confirmation of gallows humor as the solution to the impasse of the relation between life and death.

I have used the mantra of Socratic ignorance—I know that I don't know—to illustrate in part absolute humor in relation to the enigma of the Greek chorus to which I invariably must return, a refrain that seems to suggest that it is better to be ignorant and alive than to be dead! On the surface, this flies against Socrates' injunction insofar as an ignorant life is definitely to be damned. Yet this might disclose a limit of Socrates, for example in his failure to show absolute humor in his practice of inquiry, that his absolutism always risks dissolving into supercilious irony and so, might undermine his capacity to be comedic in a way noted by Aristophanes, Nietzsche, Benjamin, and some few others. If it is better not to be born than to live burdened by knowledge, then to be driven to life and to living as we do, as in most cases not being able to die, then this constraint—our being burdened by ignorance and life—must be what we know. The burden of the mix, knowledge and ignorance, is exactly as Socrates says, our knowledge. If to live is to accept ignorance, such acceptance cannot resist the temptation to exist while still knowing that such existence has an inherent excess. The temptation to exist confirms the excessive character of life itself, of what escapes it or what Jullien calls its "non-coincidence" in its exceeding itself and its determination (Jullien 2016, 60) in the way Simmel says that the non-coincidence of life and form creates a collision that can be positive as well as a sign of deficiency. That this non-coincidence of life and form must occur within life is to conceive of the reversal within living, introducing contradiction into living as its driving force (see Jullien 2016, 198 on the Hegelian maneuver).

Would not "living" be defined … as the unacceptability of contenting oneself with that point, whatever it might be, or of remaining (resting) within oneself? Therefore, as passing into one's other in order to be self, or "making oneself become other to oneself," as is said when the contradiction is grasped (Jullien 2016, 198).

We have used through this work various different writers to illuminate this moderate relationship to excess as a positive restlessness essential to living with what is settled and determined and that not only includes those who want to overcome the imperative to accept conditions as settled such as the "norms," but must make reference to those even similar to the writer Zweig, who in transgressing by recognizing such a need for renewal, still risk accepting the transgressive gesture upon which he settles as itself settled.

From beginning to end we have been using the enigmatic statement of the chorus to pose the question of the temptation to exist as forceful, inscrutable, and comedic at its core by virtue of its sign of the inborn excess integral to life that can only remain unintelligible to and for life as a mark of its transcendence as an "object." Socrates does not truly seem to appreciate the humor in such a situation because his absolutistic belief in his formula of Socratic ignorance seems to deflect him in practice from recognizing the force of the temptation to exist as itself a sign of the essential excess of life itself. As Aristophanes suggests, Socrates does not seem to give pleasure with his humor and in fact only appears funny to his admirers, possibly exemplifying the ordinary humor closer to satire rather than absolute humor. To actually practice Socratic ignorance, one would need to treat the temptation to exist seriously enough to appreciate its comedic character and this would lead to an alternative to admonishing, perhaps by representing in story the character who admonishes in a way that mixes both sides of humor in the situation of the character. This is precisely what Plato took up in his project in representing Socrates as the fool.

In this respect, we might ask whether or not the clown might be an alternative to the fool. Delpech-Ramey treats such a burden, being driven to exist, as the fate of the clown: "What the clown would like most is to be able to die. But death is precisely what is denied them" (Delpech-Ramey 2011, 133). The drive of the clown to exist while wanting to escape, that is, to live in ignorance while knowing this and this alone, is human material for travesty as a gesture that exaggerates absorption in the incidentals of life, demonstrating theatrically how what we most want to do is simultaneously that from which we want to escape; this tension between concentration and flight reveals the clown as the performer whose use of the grave incidentals of life has to entertain both oneself and the others, intending to show the lightness of being in which the performer absorbs oneself and tries to give pleasure to the other. Accordingly, when Heraclitus advises us not to imitate him but the logos, he points to this conclusion: the logos seems to mark the inherent excess in humanity or what Delpech-Ramey calls "the excessive character of life itself." This impasse, reflecting "the desire to exist beyond every limitation" reveals the transcendence not of the subject but of any "object" and its excess. The logos is then not identical to reason or the order of rationality but mixed somewhat as the need and desire to participate in a discursive relation of life to form: Heraclitus counsels us to imitate the excess inherent in life by accepting the need and delight of demonstrating being part of and apart from such a movement in practice.

Conclusion

The temptation to exist includes the temptation to be discursive in the best (poetic) sense as our opportunity in any present and must include the aged, their caregivers and anyone and everyone else. If we resist playing Sisyphus or the zombie, we can orient to our choice between Socrates and Harpo Marx, or perhaps the Chinese sage but only as the desire for the awakening T.J. Clark described in his analysis of Pouisson's paintings and that we find in Heraclitus (see Jullien 2016, 272). As a practice, awakening tries to re-achieve innocence in any present by resisting the idea that a condition, even death and the loss of life that it signals, is predetermined to be as typified by the system we inhabit, disclosing how the inborn excess of humanity always remains capable of motivating us to dream, to rise above such expectations by an effort of thought and action that can see an end as something other.

> This means not only thinking about mobility against the immutable … or about ambiguity against excess, both of which are no longer signs of lack or deficiency, but still, more generally, in thinking about the "innocence" of a "living" liberated from all external recuperation and submission to ends … we only begin to perceive "what" living is when life is already withdrawing into ourselves, through old age or sickness, and not when it rises in power or spreads out in maturity.
>
> (Jullien 2016, 167, 57)

References

Blum, Alan. 1996. "Fear and Panic: On the Phenomenology of Desperation." *The Sociological Quarterly* 37 (4): 673–699.

——. 2011. *The Grey Zone of Health and Illness*. Bristol: Intellect Press.

Baltes, Paul, and Margaret Baltes, eds. 1990. *Successful Aging Perspectives from the Behavioral Sciences*. Cambridge, MA: MIT Press.

Beaujour, Michel. 1981. "Some Paradoxes of Description." *Yale French Review* 6: 27–59.

Benjamin, Walter. 1998. *The Origin of German Tragic Drama*. Translated by John Osborne. London: Verso.

Delpech-Ramey, Joshua. 2011. "On The Inhuman Rights of Clowns." *Substance* 39 (2): 131–141.

Dillaway, Heather. 2009. "Reconsidering Successful Aging." *Journal of Applied Gerontology* 28 (6): 702–722.

Goffman, Erving. 1952. "On Cooling the Mark Out: Some Aspects of Adaptation to Failure." *Psychiatry* 15 (4): 451–463.

Jullien, Francois. 2016. *The Philosophy of Living*. Translated by Micheal Richardson and Krzysztof Fijalkowski. New York: Seagull Books.

Marder, Elissa. 2013. "Real Dreams." *The Southern Journal of Philosophy* 51. Spindel Supplement: 196–213.

Perniola, Mario. (2000) 2004. *The Sex Appeal of the Inorganic: Philosophies of Desire in the Modern World*. Translated by Massimo Verdicchio. New York and London: Continuum.

Plato. 1941. *The Republic*. Translated with an introduction and notes by F. M. Cornford. London: Oxford University Press.

Scary, Elaine. 1995. "On Vivacity: The Difference between Daydreaming and Imagining Under Authorial Instruction." *representations* 52: 1–26.

Simmel, Georg. 1971. "The Adventurer." In *On Individuality and Social Forms*. Chicago: University of Chicago Press.

Swanson, Guy. 1971. *Social Change*. London: Scott, Foresman & Company.

Weber, Max. (1921–1922) 1947. *The Theory of Social and Economic Organization*. Translated by A.M. Henderson and Talcott Parsons. New York: The Free Press.

Zupančič, Alenka. 2008. *The Odd One In: On Comedy*. Cambridge, MA: The MIT Press.

Zweig, Stefan. (1927) 2012. *Confusion*. Introduction by George Prochnik, Trans. Atheas Bell, New York: New York Review of Books.

Index

For Product Safety Concerns and Information please contact our EU representative GPSR@taylorandfrancis.com
Taylor & Francis Verlag GmbH, Kaufingerstraße 24, 80331 München, Germany

www.ingramcontent.com/pod-product-compliance
Ingram Content Group UK Ltd.
Pitfield, Milton Keynes, MK11 3LW, UK
UKHW022130190926
475702UK00013B/1730
9780367224042